# AROMATHERAPY FOR NATURAL LIVING

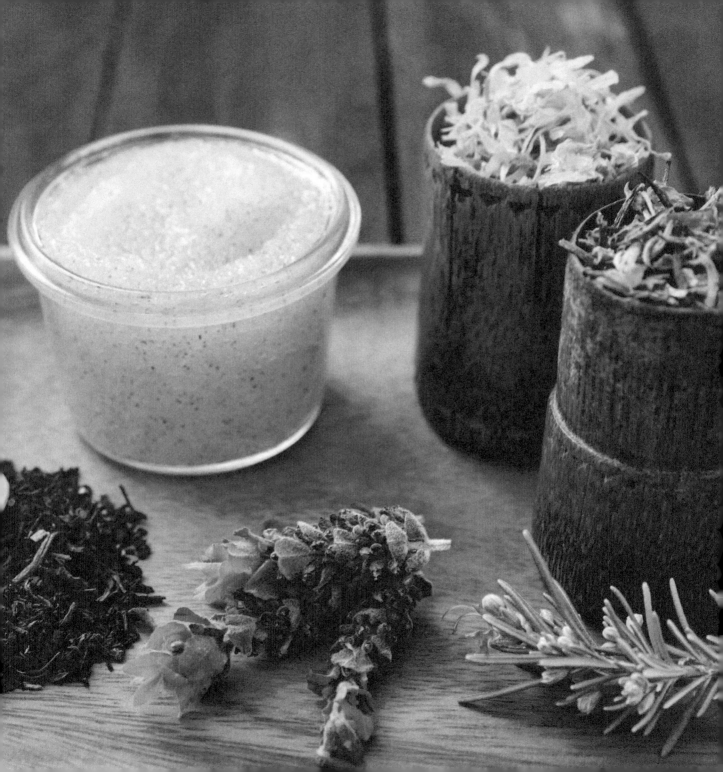

# Aromatherapy
## *for Natural Living*

— THE A–Z REFERENCE —

*of* ESSENTIAL OILS REMEDIES *for* HEALTH, BEAUTY *and* THE HOME

ANNE KENNEDY

ALTHEA
PRESS

# CONTENTS

## FIVE Aromatherapy Recipes for Beauty 237

## SIX Aromatherapy Recipes for the Home 289

# SEVEN Essential Oil Profiles *341*

# INTRODUCTION

After a particularly stressful period in my life, a concerned friend introduced me to aromatherapy. I was initially skeptical, but I quickly discovered lavender essential oil's ability to produce a feeling of relaxation and to promote the peaceful sleep I so desperately needed. After making this initial connection, I was fascinated. Naturally, I wanted to know more. Over the past ten years, I have studied the principles of English and French aromatherapy and put them into practice. I use essential oils to make fragrant potions for natural skin care, to formulate wonderful, nontoxic household cleaners and pet products, and to support my health and that of my loved ones. Aromatherapy makes my daily life more pleasant, and I love to share what I've learned with others.

You're holding this book because you, too, have an interest in aromatherapy, and you want to know more. Perhaps you're wondering why you keep seeing essential oils available at places other than health food stores. Maybe you have enjoyed an aromatherapy treatment or two at your favorite spa, and perhaps you've even tried popular essential oils like lavender or peppermint at home.

You might already know that essential oils are very different from other treatments, and you may have heard anecdotes from friends or family members who are overjoyed by the benefits they have received from these effective, easy-to-use natural remedies. There's a lot to learn about aromatherapy—but before you begin, you should know that it's gaining popularity not just because essential oils smell so good, but because they really do work!

Some believe aromatherapy offers benefits beyond those found in the chemical composition of essential oils. While there might be something to those beliefs, there is nothing mystical about aromatherapy. Aromatherapy offers health benefits because of the essential oils' chemical structure, components of which include terpenes, oxides, esters, alcohols, ketones, phenols, and aldehydes. These substances are so effective that they are also used in pharmaceuticals. You'll learn more about them in chapter 2.

The "aroma" part of aromatherapy explains the first way essential oils can make their way into your system—through your sense of smell. The second way is through your skin, which is a permeable membrane. When you apply a

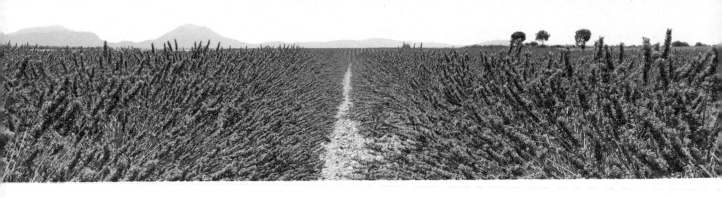

treatment made with essential oils topically, the oils are absorbed directly into the tissues beneath the skin's surface, where they perform specific actions such as increasing circulation or numbing pain. Of course, we're just skimming the surface. You'll find a concise explanation of the science of aromatherapy in chapter 2.

While some advocate for treating ailments by taking essential oils by mouth, remedies that call for ingestion are outside the realm of aromatherapy in home practice and should take place only under professional supervision. For this reason, and because the nature of essential oils can change during the digestive process, the remedies found within these pages are meant to be applied topically or inhaled.

If you're looking for a way to cut back your intake of pain relievers or tackle insomnia without resorting to a prescription sleep aid, aromatherapy can help. Essential oils provide natural relief for common ailments like headaches and colds, along with less-common problems like exposure to poison ivy. This book contains remedies for more than 90 ailments, plus wonderful aromatherapy treatments for bath and beauty. Finally, you'll find 25 ways to use essential oils around the house, with fragrant alternatives to chemical-laden cleaning solutions, laundry detergents, and more.

You can easily cut back on chemicals by selecting just a handful of the 85 essential oils described in this book. Add a few more, and you'll find that you depend on commercial products far less than before. When you formulate your own aromatherapy treatments, you ultimately save money, reduce your exposure to toxins, and take charge of your health naturally. By supporting your well-being with aromatherapy, you'll do more than just delight your senses; you'll enhance your entire lifestyle.

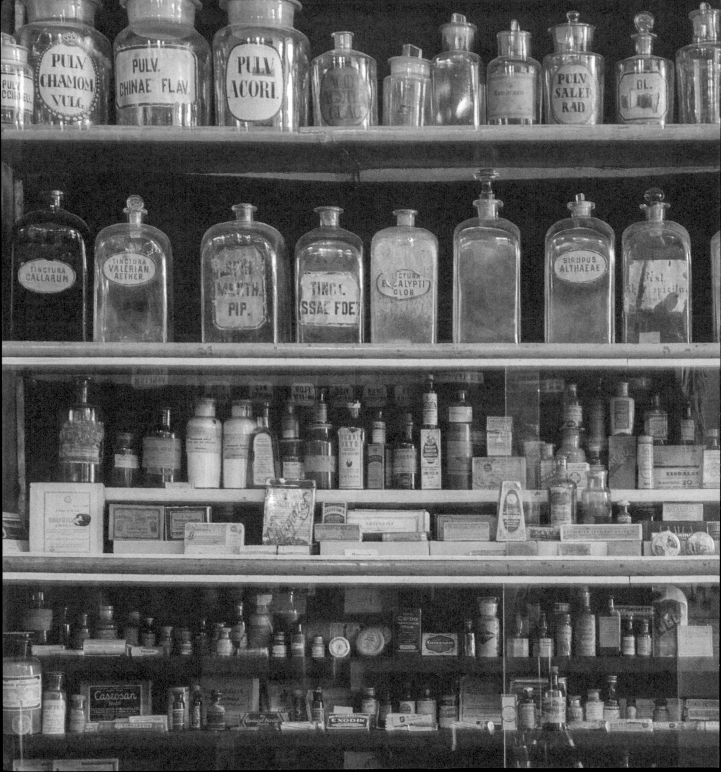

# ONE

# Rooted in History

The essential oils that make up today's aromatherapy treatments are rooted in thousands of years of history. It's likely that humankind began using of aromatic herbs—even for simple enjoyment—long before recorded history. In this chapter, we'll travel back through time, and you'll see how our ancestors developed fragrant, plant-based remedies to promote health and hygiene.

## Why Aromatherapy?

What is aromatherapy and what are some of its benefits? At its most fundamental, aromatherapy is exactly what it sounds like: the use of volatile plant extracts, especially essential oils, in treatments designed to promote physical and psychological well-being. You might be wondering about the term *volatile*. In aromatherapy, this word refers to essential oils' tendency to evaporate rapidly.

As you'll soon discover, aromatherapy isn't just about essential oils. Treatments can include complementary ingredients like pre-diluted essential oils such as rose and jasmine, rich emollients like nut oils and beeswax, healing herbs and herbal extracts, milk powders, sugars, pure sea salts, muds, and clays.

What you won't find in true aromatherapy treatments are synthetic ingredients such as perfume oils or fragrance oils made with chemicals. These oils may smell similar to essential oils, but they don't provide any therapeutic benefits, and they might even cause unpleasant side effects such as headaches, hives, or nausea.

The essential oils in holistic aromatherapy treatments offer many physical, mental, and emotional benefits, helping you achieve better health, greater beauty, and improved hygiene. Long before laboratories and pharmacies, people relied on plants for well-being. And although the term *aromatherapy* came into use during the twentieth century, its foundations date back to ancient times. We'll be taking a closer look at historical uses of aromatherapy in the next section.

## Benefits of Aromatherapy

Aromatherapy provides many benefits, and as you'll learn in chapter 7, each essential oil offers different properties. The following list outlines some examples of the many ways you can use aromatherapy to enhance your well-being.

**Boost energy levels**  Whether you're trying to cut back on caffeine or looking for a way to keep your energy level up during long workdays, you'll find that aromatherapy offers a variety of fragrant solutions. Many essential oils increase circulation, gently stimulating your body and mind without causing any unpleasant side effects. Peppermint, black pepper, and cinnamon leaf are some examples.

**Change cognitive states**  Anxiousness, nervousness, and other negative emotions are difficult to deal with, especially when they happen frequently. The essential oils used in aromatherapy have a direct impact on the brain's emotional center, and they can provide rapid relief from troublesome thought processes. Lavender and basil both address anxiousness, and rose oil helps decrease stress.

**Eliminate headaches**  You don't have to rely on potentially toxic drugs to obtain headache relief; a number of essential oils can help. Lavender is one of them; it has been proven to alleviate migraines. Peppermint and spearmint are two others that work well.

**Enhance memory**  Scents and memories are closely intertwined, and some essential oils have the ability to improve memory. Rosemary has been proven to improve cognitive learning and decrease the amount of time it takes students to answer test questions correctly.

**Heighten immunity**  You may already know that good nutrition boosts your immune system; aromatherapy works in a similar way, by making cells strong and healthy so that they are better at fighting disease when needed. Bergamot, lavender, and tea tree are just a few examples of essential oils that stimulate the immune system.

**Improve mood**  Moods such as sadness, anger, and irritation can hide under the surface and take the joy out of life. Aromatherapy makes a positive difference in a variety of ways; for example, jasmine has a direct, positive effect on the limbic system, which is directly linked to mood, and lemon increases norepinephrine, which in turn provides an immediate mood boost.

**Nourish skin** Many aromatherapy recipes call for rich, moisturizing carrier oils and creams, and essential oils themselves help improve skin. Just like the plants they come from, essential oils like lavender and helichrysum contain vitamins and antioxidants, which nourish the skin on a cellular level.

**Promote healing** Many plants have the power to help the body heal faster: Because essential oils are highly concentrated, they can have an impressive healing effect. Helichrysum, for example, offers strong anti-inflammatory action, and it contains regenerative molecules that facilitate skin's ability to knit itself back together following an injury.

**Provide stress relief** Stress is a normal response to life's challenges, but that doesn't mean you have to live with it. Most aromatherapy treatments are a pleasure to use, and that alone can help you feel less stressed. Some essential oils have been studied for their ability to reduce stress; frankincense, for example, contains sesquiterpenes that cross the blood-brain barrier and stimulate the limbic system, immediately calming the mind and making it easier to deal with difficult emotions.

**Relieve discomfort** Aspirin and acetaminophen are two examples of analgesics—substances that stop pain. Many essential oils, such as tagetes and rosewood, also offer analgesic properties, and they often make suitable substitutes for over-the-counter medications. Sunburns, paper cuts, and minor sprains are just a few examples of painful problems that respond well to aromatherapy.

## Historical Background

The term *aromatherapy* was coined in the 1920s by a French chemist, René-Maurice Gattefossé, who suffered a terrible burn in a laboratory accident. After applying lavender essential oil to cool the burn, he was astonished to discover that his injury healed quickly and without scarring. Gattefossé, however, wasn't the first to discover the healing power of concentrated plant oils. Cave paintings in Sibudu Cave, located in South Africa near Richards Bay, reveal that medicinal plants with insecticidal and larvicidal properties played an important role in the daily life of prehistoric humans. These paintings date back to about 75,000 BCE.

Ancient Greeks, Romans, Persians, and Egyptians used medicinal plants, as did Chinese physicians and many others. Evidence and recorded history show that Egyptians were using aromatic oils from as early as 4500 BCE onward, transforming them into ointments, suppositories, medicinal cakes, powders, and pills.

## ANCIENT EGYPT

The Ebers Papyrus, a scroll dating back to about 1500 BCE, details more than 800 remedies using herbs and aromatic oils. And, when archaeologists opened King Tut's tomb in 1922, they found 50 alabaster jars for holding oils, including frankincense.

In ancient Egypt, herbal preparations and infused oils were used for medicinal, spiritual, cosmetic, and fragrant use. Egyptians used a good deal of incense, and they used plant oils including cedarwood, cinnamon leaf, clove, myrrh, galbanum, spikenard, and nutmeg in funeral rites and mummification rituals. Many of these precious herbs and spices were laboriously transported across vast stretches of desert, usually by Middle Eastern merchants who also traveled to Assyria, Babylon, China, Greece, Rome, and Persia. This was such a popular route that it became known as the Frankincense Trail.

Typically depicted as elegant, well-coiffed figures, ancient Egyptian women weren't the only ones who appreciated fine fragrances. Egyptian men loved them, too; in fact, people of both genders wore cones of solidified perfumed oil on their heads, which would release fragrances as the cones gradually melted. It's no surprise then that Egyptian ancients are credited with the creation of the word *perfume*, which comes from the Latin words *per fumum*. This literally translates as "through smoke."

They believed that as the smoke of fragrant incense rose to the heavens, it would honor their gods and carry their wishes and prayers up for consideration. Interestingly, incense is still used in spiritual rites today, with many mainstream and alternative religions continuing the tradition.

Ancient Egyptians are also credited with the invention of a machine for distilling cedarwood oil. Made of terra-cotta and dated to 3000 BCE, it was discovered during a 1975 archaeological expedition led by Dr. Paolo Rovesti. It is believed that scientists in ancient India and Persia may have created distillation machines of their own, but little is known about how or when these tools came into use.

## ANCIENT GREECE AND ROME

In 2003, archaeologists discovered what appeared to be an ancient perfume factory on the Mediterranean island of Cyprus inside a larger industrial complex in the city of Pyrgos. Inside, they found clay alembic stills dating to about 2000 BCE, along with perfume bottles and mixing jugs. (An alembic still is a three-part distilling apparatus.) Upon analysis, 14 botanical residues were discovered, along with four recipes for making perfumes.

Ancient Greeks learned many of their healing techniques from the Egyptians, using herbs and oils for cosmetics, medicines, and fine fragrances. Asclepius, circa 800 BCE, is known to have experimented with plants and herbs.

His impact as a healer was so profound that he was deified after his death and is known today as the god of healing in Greek mythology. Another famous figure was a perfumer called Megallus, who created a signature perfume known as Megaleion. Like other perfumes of the day, it had an oil base and relied on myrrh to provide a pleasing aroma. What made it unusual was that Megaleion didn't just smell nice; it was also used to heal wounds and improve skin.

Hippocrates, known as the father of medicine, was active around 400 BCE and studied hundreds of botanicals for their benefits. He believed that they could be used not just to promote good health, but also to prevent more invasive treatments. He often used fennel, parsley, valerian, and hypericum in his treatments.

We have Hippocrates to thank not just for the serious, formal study of medicine, but for being among the first to believe that the physical body, mind, and spirit are interconnected parts of an organism. This theory is called *holism* and is one of the concepts fundamental to the practices of aromatherapy and holistic medicine.

Theophrastus and Pedanius Dioscorides are famous among the many Greek physicians who dealt primarily with herbs and aromatic oils. Dioscorides is known for serving in Nero's army. As the army marched through Greece, Spain, Italy, and Germany, Dioscorides recorded every plant and mineral he discovered. He collected specimens, described

habitats, and gave full accounts of their healing properties in the five-volume work, *De Materia Medica*. This massive resource describes well over 500 plants and aromatics, including familiar ones such as marjoram, basil, dill, jasmine, and cinnamon, in stunning detail. The entire *Dioscorea* genus of plants, which includes familiar species such as the yam, was named after Dioscorides.

The Romans further developed Egyptian and Greek techniques for distilling aromatic remedies, and they took great advantage of their predecessors' natural medical knowledge. The Greeks' understanding continued to advance: around 150 CE, physician Claudius Galenus (also known as Galen) used his extensive knowledge of medicinal herbs and plants to treat hundreds of injured gladiators. Later, he became the personal physician of the Roman emperor Marcus Aurelius.

Galen was brilliant and influential; he was also the last great Greco-Roman physician. Within 100 years of his passing, the Roman Empire began to decline, and Europe was swiftly plunged into the Dark Ages.

## MIDDLE EAST

Middle Eastern history provides insight into the region's role in aromatherapy's history. During a 1975 archaeological expedition to Pakistan's Indus Valley, Dr. Paolo Rovesti viewed a terra-cotta device and several terra-cotta perfume containers in a museum. These were similar to a still that was dated 3000 BCE, about 4,000 years earlier than the official date of the invention of distillation. A similar vessel was discovered in Afghanistan.

The Epic of Gilgamesh discusses how the King of Ur (a part of Mesopotamia located in present-day Iraq) burned incense to please the gods and goddesses. In neighboring Babylonia, a tablet that dates back to about 2700 BCE contains an order for the import of aromatics including cedar, cypress, and myrrh.

Middle Eastern trade routes were used extensively, with aromatic goods being a valuable part of many shipments. The Old Testament describes one group of traders as a "company of Ishmaelites [Arabs] from Gilead, bearing spicery, balm, and myrrh, going to carry it down to Egypt." As early as 1500 BCE, double-outrigger canoes were used to carry spices from Southeast Asia to the Middle East, following pathways known as maritime spice routes. The cinnamon route crossed the Indian Ocean to Africa, whereas the clove route hugged the coastline.

Persian physician Muhammad ibn Zakariya al-Razi was born between 854 and 862 CE, near the area now known as Tehran. Over his lifetime, he penned 237 known books and articles that detail various aspects of science, with about half of those covering the medicinal use of plants. He didn't just write and practice medicine; he invented a number of important medical tools, including vials, spatulas, flasks, and mortars, that made working with plants easier. Many of his designs were used in pharmacies until they were replaced with modern iterations during the early twentieth century.

Around 1000 CE, Persian physician Ibn Sina (also known as Avicenna) invented a coiled pipe that steam-distilled plants to produce essential oils similar to the ones we enjoy today. Often referred to as the Prince of Physicians, this remarkable man wrote numerous books and treatises on medicine, including an epic 14-volume series called *Al-Qanun Fi Al-Tibb*, or *The Canon of Medicine*. Over a million words long, it contained all medical knowledge of the day, including Galenic and Hippocratic traditions, along with his own observations. For more than 700 years, this work was regarded as the definitive medical textbook, reference, and teaching guide for the Eastern and European worlds.

## EAST AND ASIA

Aromatherapy was used throughout ancient China, with the use of aromatic oils first being recorded during the reign of Huang-ti, known as the Yellow Emperor. During this era, which lasted from about 2697 to 2597 BCE, he wrote *The Yellow Emperor's Classic of Internal Medicine*, which contains many uses for aromatics and is still in use by today's practitioners of Eastern medicine.

# AYURVEDA AND AROMATHERAPY

The Indian practice of Ayurveda, or Life Knowledge, is the oldest form of medicine, having been in continuous use for thousands of years. Even during the Dark Ages, when much knowledge was lost to the Western world, Indians continued using plants and aromatic oils therapeutically.

In Ayurveda, jasmine is used as a general tonic for the whole body. Rose is as an antidepressant and a liver strengthener. For colds, Ayurvedic practitioners recommend chamomile, which also is used in remedies for issues ranging from dizziness to headaches. Like essential oils used in aromatherapy, these plants offer multiple benefits, and practitioners view them with the same validity that Western doctors reserve for lab-created pharmaceuticals.

Vedic literature mentions more than 700 substances, many of which are frequently used in aromatherapy. Cinnamon, myrrh, ginger, and sandalwood are among them. Often, sweet and spicy aromas like cinnamon and sandalwood are blended to create a sense of calm, and cool-smelling oils such as rose and patchouli are used to clear the mind.

Basil, cedar, and sage are among the oils Ayurveda practitioners use to clear congestion, while lavender and sandalwood are among those used for fever. These are just a few examples—there are many similarities between ancient Ayurvedic practices and modern aromatherapy. To deepen your knowledge, check out *Ayurveda & Aromatherapy: The Earth Essential Guide to Ancient Wisdom and Modern Healing* (Lotus Press, 1995).

While ancient Egyptians, Greeks, Arabs, and Romans wore lots of perfumed oils and used them in baths, cosmetics, and other beauty treatments, Chinese culture emphasized the use of fragrances for purity and disinfection. The practice of burning incense in special spaces, particularly in temples, remains popular throughout many parts of Asia today.

Historians have shown that noblewomen used mandarin to scent their hands and that the period between the Sui and Song dynasties (581–1279 CE) was quite fragrant, with nobles importing ingredients via the Silk Road and competing to create the best personal scents. By the time of the Qing dynasty in 1644, the emperor carried a special perfume pouch filled with fragrant herbs. Despite a report by the *Jing Daily* stating Chinese people did not have a history of using fragrances, perfume pouches are still popular today and are given as special tokens of esteem.

## EUROPE

Christian crusaders who traveled east in search of the Holy Grail returned without the coveted cup of Christ, but with knowledge of herbal remedies. Soon, aromatics became popular in Europe.

During the twelfth century, a German abbess named Hildegard of Bingen famously wrote medicinal and botanical texts. Highly regarded for her practical applications of herbs, tinctures, and even precious stones, Abbess Hildegard catalogued her knowledge in a series of nine books called the *Physica*. A subsequent work called *Causae et Curae* explores the human body, describes its connection to the natural world, and outlines the causes of and cures for numerous diseases. Hildegard's books provide remedies for common ailments such as burns and cuts, along with methods for treating more serious injuries, including dislocations and fractures.

The thirteenth century saw the beginnings of the pharmaceutical industry, and an increase in the distillation and popularity of essential oils. Unfortunately, the medieval era also saw many Catholic leaders rejecting most medicine, believing its use showed defiance of God's just punishments. When the Black Death arrived in Sicily in 1347, plague spread through Europe like wildfire, and within five years, about one-third of the population had perished. It is believed that many herbalists and perfumers escaped illness due to their constant contact with medicinal plants and essential oils.

Various versions of an unsubstantiated, but popular, story claim that during an episode of the plague, four robbers were arrested while stripping the deceased of their valuables. The king, likely Edward III of England, offered to spare their lives if they would reveal the secret to their ability to come into close contact with plague victims without becoming ill themselves. Spice traders and perfumers by profession, the thieves said that they used a blend of clove, cinnamon, eucalyptus, lemon, and rosemary essential oils that they rubbed all over their bodies and inside the masks they breathed through. Different variations of this story state that the thieves used herbs and vinegar and that they were active in Marseilles, France. Like different versions of the story of the four thieves, a variety of recipes for "thieves' oil" remedies remains very popular today.

During the Renaissance, merchants brought rich incenses, potent herbs, and exotic natural remedies back to Europe, where they gained instant popularity. Wealthy citizens carried scented handkerchiefs or ornate pomanders with them, inhaling frequently to avoid unpleasant smells while unwittingly protecting themselves from germs. Frankincense, rose, rosemary, sage, and juniper were among the most popular scents of the era.

At the same time, pharmacists, chemists, and physicians intensified their studies of plants and began to distill essential oils on a larger scale. During the sixteenth century, herbalists and other medical practitioners built apothecaries that specialized in the production of herbals and essential oils that were used in pharmaceuticals, fragrances, and food throughout Europe. During this time, German physician, botanist, and alchemist Hieronymus Brunschwig authored books on essential oil distillation during this time, in which he notes 25 oils, including lavender, rosemary, cinnamon, clove, and nutmeg.

The connection between disease and microorganisms was made in the 1880s. In 1887, French physicians tested the antibacterial properties of essential oils following an observation that tuberculosis wasn't as common in the flower-growing districts of southern France as it was elsewhere. In 1888, scientists published a study that showed that the microorganisms responsible for glandular and yellow fever were killed by active constituents found in Chinese cinnamon, oregano, geranium, and angelica.

Perfumery had become an art form by the seventeenth century, and it remained popular during the eighteenth century. By the nineteenth century, wealthy women had their jewelers craft fine bottles to hold signature scents. Something else happened during the nineteenth century: major essential oils' constituents were isolated, and chemical drugs based on "active ingredients" were put into production. Knowledge grew, and during the twentieth century, laboratory workers were able to create synthetic chemicals and pharmaceuticals that mimicked those found in natural plant matter. These discoveries led to synthetic fragrances, as well as to medicine as we now know it, and essential oils took a backseat to these new discoveries.

## Modern Aromatherapy

Remember René-Maurice Gattefossé, the chemist who was burned while working in his lab? He went on to use his knowledge to treat burns, gangrene, skin infections, and soldiers' wounds throughout World War I. In 1928, he coined the term *aromatherapy* in an article that supported the use of whole essential oils rather than individual, chemically isolated components. In 1937, he wrote a highly regarded book, *Gattefossé's Aromatherapy*, which is still in print.

Aromatherapy experienced a renaissance in the twentieth century with Jean Valnet, MD, Madame Marguerite Maury, and author Robert Tisserand emerging as experts in the field.

Dr. Valnet, author of *The Practice of Aromatherapy*, used essential oils including clove, chamomile, lemon, and thyme to treat soldiers wounded during World War II. He is also known as the first person to treat psychiatric conditions with aromatherapy. Madame Marguerite Maury, a biochemist, avidly studied, practiced, and passed on her knowledge of aromatherapy, using essential oils and complementary substances primarily for their cosmetic benefits. And, in 1977, English aromatherapist Robert B. Tisserand published his famous book, *The Art of Aromatherapy*. It remains highly regarded to this day.

## THE 1980S

Today's awareness of aromatherapy began with a resurgence of interest that started in the 1970s and gained momentum in the 1980s. Dr. Valnet played a leading role, expanding his theories in numerous books, publications, and medical journals.

Aromatherapy was first popular in Europe, where it remains a mainstay today. The practice took longer to catch on in the United States. Slowly but surely, herbalists, homeopaths, and natural health therapists began to see increasing interest in their endeavors, and schools and colleges began to offer a wider range of massage therapy courses. People all over the world began to regain trust in natural remedies and slowly started to use aromatherapy to complement Western medicine.

## AROMATHERAPY TODAY

Today, we have the privilege of unfettered access to knowledge, and in many places, aromatherapy is a household word. Even people who have never benefitted from it are interested in learning more and are eager to try essential oils for themselves. People are once again beginning to look toward self-healing, and medical professionals are coming to recognize the important complementary role that aromatherapy can play.

As you'll learn in the next chapter, the science behind aromatherapy is sound. Holistic health practitioners, naturopaths, acupuncturists, traditional Chinese medical practitioners, chiropractors, and a growing number of hospitals and cancer treatment centers offer aromatherapy treatments. Sometimes presented as an alternative form of medicine, they are more often offered in complementary treatments designed to alleviate stress and anxiety.

# MODERN AROMATHERAPY OUTSIDE THE UNITED STATES

Outside the United States, aromatherapy is more accepted by mainstream medical practitioners as something more than simple, supportive care for improving life quality. In France and Japan, for example, medical aromatherapy is a well-established field that addresses conditions ranging from diabetes to seizure disorders.

French, British, and German schools of thought hold different standards and goals for the medical use of aromatherapy, so it's easy to become confused when learning what essential oils are best for and how they are used.

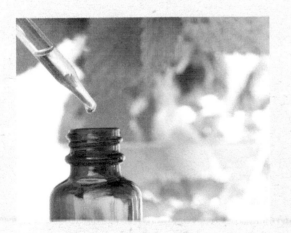

British aromatherapy ideals are closest to those promoted and practiced in America, with most essential oils being heavily diluted before application and no ingestion of essential oil remedies. French methods focus on applying essential oils undiluted (neat), as well as using some oils internally. Both models encourage inhalation.

Medical doctors in France and Germany dispense aromatherapy treatments, including those that call for the ingestion of encapsulated essential oils. In France, where medical aromatherapy is very popular, doctors use a laboratory technique called the *aromatogram*, in which cultures from patients' infections are exposed to various essential oils to find the one that best treats that specific infection.

Despite their differences, professional aromatherapy practitioners everywhere are quick to convey the importance of using high-quality essential oils from trusted sources for all treatments. Whether you are applying aromatherapy treatments topically or using them for inhalation, it's important to give your body the best, purest oils.

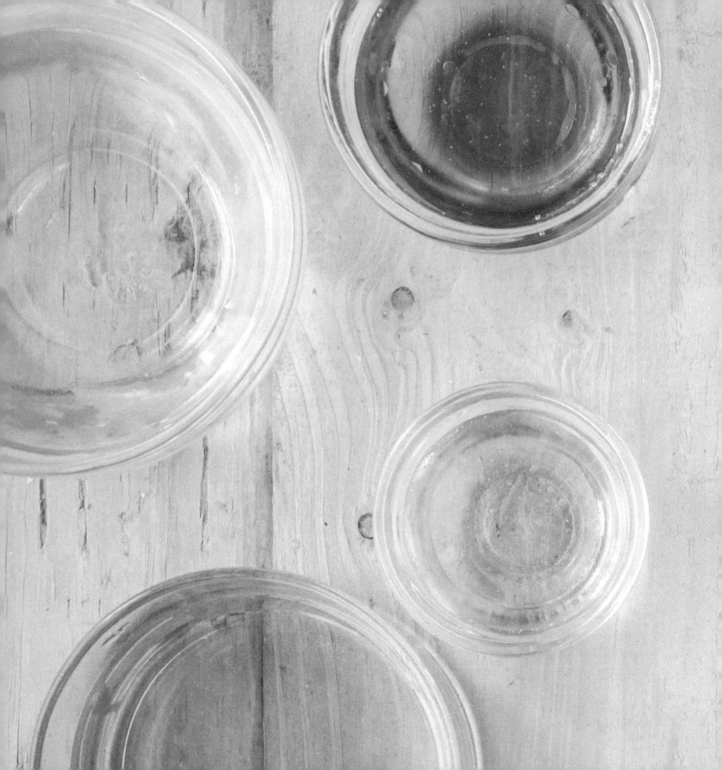

# TWO

# Rooted in Science

The history of aromatherapy is just that—history. It is in the present we find research and documentation of aromatherapy's benefits. While much of what we know about aromatherapy has its roots planted firmly in the fertile soil of the past, scientific evidence often supports treatments and provides insight into how and why aromatherapy works.

## Behind the Scents

We've got the history down, but how does aromatherapy actually work? All of the following are involved in the inner workings of aromatherapy:

### IT BEGINS WITH YOUR NOSE

The nose serves as a direct link from the world around us to the brain, and the knowledge of whether certain things smell good or bad is partly built in. For example, when we smell something burning unexpectedly, we feel a sense of urgency. Alternately, when we smell food cooking at mealtimes, the stomach responds with hungry growls. Other smells are directly connected to emotions. The crisp scent of freshly mowed grass, the clean tang of salty sea air, and the sweet aroma of holiday treats baking in the oven are examples of smells that transport us back to times when we experienced some of life's most memorable moments.

The incredible sense of smell works when any substance with a scent emits molecules into the air. When the nose picks up the molecules, it transports them past the trigeminal nerve receptors, which are responsible for guarding the olfactory system by sensing irritants and triggering sneezes that eject the offending molecules. Molecules that make their way past these guard cells are taken up by nasal mucus, where they are dissolved before being transported through tiny olfactory receptor cells in the epithelium, the thin tissue that lines the outer layer of hollow body structures.

Once olfactory receptor cells are activated, they signal the olfactory bulb, which is the part of the brain's structure located above the nasal cavity, directly beneath the frontal lobe. Next, the receptor cells synapse on the second-order neurons that form the olfactory tract, and the scent's signal travels further into the brain, where it synapses with cells in the amygdala and prepiriform cortex before traveling to the hypothalamus and other parts of the brain.

The sections of the brain that receive scent signals are directly involved in emotional control, memory recall, immune function, hormone production, basic drives, and more. Aromas can alter your heart rate, blood pressure, and breath rate. They can also stimulate the release of beta-endorphins, including endogenous opioids, which are the body's natural mood elevators and painkillers. These peptides are responsible for creating the euphoria or "runner's high" following a great workout.

There is nothing—not even an advanced drug—you can take orally that affects your brain as quickly as scent will. And, if you inhale via both nose and mouth, molecules will quickly enter your lungs and make their way into your bloodstream.

## AND GETS UNDER YOUR SKIN . . .

Aromatherapy isn't just about fragrance; it's also about the effect essential oils have when they come in contact with your skin. If you're familiar with transdermal patches like those used to deliver nicotine to people trying to quit tobacco, then you already have a good idea how topical aromatherapy treatments work. Like those found in nicotine patches, the molecules in essential oils are capable of transdermal action, penetrating the skin and rapidly making their way through the entire body.

## THEN IMPACTS YOUR CELLS . . .

Because they are made up of tiny molecules, essential oils are capable of crossing through tissue and cell walls easily. These microscopic molecules are so minuscule that they're even able to cross through the blood-brain barrier, a filtering mechanism that blocks the passage of certain substances into the brain. No wonder they work so quickly!

Once an aromatherapy treatment's active essential oil molecules get into your cells, they perform some specific functions. Some treatments support the digestive, endocrine, circulatory, nervous, or reproductive systems, and some provide defense against bacteria and viruses.

Many essential oils are also powerful antioxidants with the ability to cleanse the cells of harmful free radicals that form as part of the natural metabolic process, as well as those that enter the body via external sources such as cigarette smoke, air pollution, or exposure to chemicals. Because free radicals can damage cells, it's important to treat your body to plenty of antioxidants. Colorful vegetables and fruits are also a great source, so eating right and using aromatherapy in place of chemical-laden products can be an important part of a solid foundation for defending your health.

## Producing Essential Oils

The essential oils at the heart of aromatherapy treatments are produced via a few key methods. Some are centuries or even millennia old; others are new, highly technical procedures.

### DISTILLATION

The process of distillation dates back thousands of years, but it's such an effective way to obtain essential oils that its use continues today. In fact, steam distillation remains the most popular of all essential oil production methods.

The steam distillation process begins when plant material is placed inside a sealed still. Pressurized water vapor travels through the chamber and slowly breaks down the plant matter. As the steam rises up through a connecting pipe that leads to a condenser, it carries with it the rapidly evaporating molecules—that is, the volatile constituents of the plant material.

The condenser cools the steam and the volatile constituents back into liquid form, and the liquid is collected in a chamber located under the condenser. Because oil does not mix with water, the essential oil floats on the water's surface or, depending on type, sinks to the bottom of the chamber. The essential oil is siphoned off and bottled, and the water, which is called hydrosol, is often reserved for use in fragrances.

While the steam distillation method previously discussed is most widely used, there are some other similar distillation processes for producing essential oils. In water distillation, plant materials—particularly delicate flowers—come into direct contact with the water. In a related process called water and steam distillation, the plant material is placed on a grate above a chamber of water, from which steam rises. The steam pressure is lower than that used in standard steam distillation, and the process takes more time to complete.

## SOLVENT EXTRACTION

Solvent extraction is used to obtain essential oils called absolutes, which come from aromatic plant materials that are too fragile for distillation. This method calls for the use of solvents like ethanol, hexane, methanol, or petroleum ether, which are used to create an extract called a concrete. The concrete contains waxes and fats from the plant matter, along with its odiferous constituents. After being mixed with alcohol, the concrete yields absolute, which is mostly aromatic oil, but contains a very low concentration of residual solvent; in most cases, it is less than 0.0001%, or 10 parts per million.

Solvent extraction is a costly process, and only a handful of aromatherapy oils are produced using this method. They include rose, jasmine, orange blossom, gardenia, and violet leaf, along with some others.

## ENFLEURAGE

Enfleurage is another method for producing absolutes. While it's not common, you might encounter costly florals such as jasmine and tuberose that have been extracted this way. In enfleurage, animal or vegetable fat is combined with freshly picked petals, which are left in the fat for a period of time that ranges from days to weeks. The petals are removed from the fat after the allotted amount of time has passed, and the process is repeated until the original fat is completely saturated with essential oil.

The resulting product is called *enfleurage pomade*. It is washed with alcohol, which separates the essential oil from the original fat. The fat retains the fragrance of the petals and is used to make soap.

## EXPRESSION

Also known as cold pressing, expression is used to produce citrus essential oils including bergamot, mandarin, lime, and sweet orange. Originally accomplished by a labor-intensive hand-pressing process, it is now accomplished via a machine-pressing process called *ecuelle à piquer*.

Citrus rinds are first placed in a rotating chamber, where they are pricked and prodded. The resulting essential oil flows into a second chamber located beneath the first one. After collection, the collection chamber spins, and centrifugal force separates the pure oil from any remaining water or fruit juice.

## HYPERCRITICAL $CO_2$ EXTRACTION

Hypercritical $CO_2$ extraction employs carbon dioxide, which is pressurized to bring it to a liquid state. Liquefied carbon dioxide is an inert solvent that is mixed with plant matter. As the pressure is released and the liquid $CO_2$ returns to its gaseous state, pure essential oil is left behind. Essential

# MAKE YOUR OWN ESSENTIAL OILS

If you grow lots of organic lavender, peppermint, or other plants popularly used in aromatherapy, you might be interested in making your own essential oils. There are a few different types of stills for home use; prices range from just over $100 to thousands of dollars. It's also possible to produce a little bit of essential oil for personal use even without a still. These typically retain freshness for six months to a year, plus they have a lovely scent and are fun to make. Here's how:

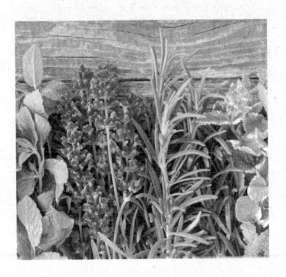

1. Fill a slow cooker to the brim with fresh, organic plant material. For lavender, use flowers, stems, and leaves; for mint, use the leaves and stems.

2. Fill the slow cooker to the top with distilled water and top it with its lid. Select the lowest setting and cook the herbs for 24 hours.

3. Remove the lid from the slow cooker and use a brand-new turkey baster to carefully siphon the essential oil from the water's surface. You can strain the plant matter from the aromatic water if you like, and use the water as linen or room spray. The water will remain fresh for about a week or two when refrigerated; use it while it lasts!

4. Transfer the essential oil into a dark-colored glass bottle and cover the bottle's mouth with cheesecloth, securing it with twine or a rubber band.

5. Allow the bottle to sit for a week so that any water inside will evaporate. Cap the bottle tightly and store it in a cool, dark place between uses.

oils produced via this method are usually a bit more expensive than their traditionally distilled counterparts, but they may contain some elements not found in traditional products from the same plants, and their aroma is often close to that of the source plant. For example, frankincense $CO_2$ extract offers anti-inflammatory and immune-enhancing properties not found in steam-distilled frankincense essential oil. On the other hand, $CO_2$ extracts from plants that aren't organically grown might contain traces of pesticide, which isn't beneficial. If you're thinking about buying $CO_2$ extracted essential oils, it's best to conduct some research on the products you are considering before making your purchase.

## Chemistry 101

What follows is a rundown of the chemical compounds that make up many of your favorite essential oils. While this is by no means an extensive lesson in organic chemistry, it will provide you with additional insight into the way aromatherapy works. For an in-depth study, I recommend *The Chemistry of Aromatherapeutic Oils* by E. Joy Bowles. This is one of the most comprehensive resources available at the time of this writing.

**Alcohols**  Alcohols are highly preservative, with the ability to resist damage from oxidation. They offer strong antibacterial action, and

are antifungal and antiviral as well. Geranium, lavender, and tea tree are some examples of essential oils with a high percentage of alcohol.

**Esters**  An ester is the result of an alcohol combining with an acid. Essential oils that contain a high percentage of esters are often quite calming and relaxing. Examples include valerian, German chamomile, Roman chamomile, and bergamot.

**Ketones**  Ketones are carbon-based compounds that often possess calming or sedative properties. Essential oils with high ketone content are excellent for expelling mucus, and they stimulate cellular regeneration. Examples include rosemary, hyssop, and western red cedar.

**Monoterpenes**  Also known as monoterpene alcohols, monoterpenes provide antiseptic, antifungal, and antiviral effects, usually without irritating skin. Citronella, lavender, and juniper are some examples of monoterpene-rich essential oils.

**Oxides**  When other chemical compounds are oxidized, the result is an oxide. Oxides often come from terpenes, alcohols, and ketones. They are a good choice for expelling mucus that accompanies a cold or flu, and can be mildly stimulating. Examples include eucalyptus, ravensara leaf, and rosemary.

**Phenols** Phenols are oxygenated compounds, including carvacrol, eugenol, and thymol. Phenols are antiseptics, but they are strong enough to irritate skin and mucous membranes. Cinnamon, clove, and wintergreen are some examples of highly phenolic essential oils.

**Sesquiterpenes** Also known as sesquiterpene alcohols, sesquiterpenes are less common than many other essential oil components. Their anti-allergen and anti-inflammatory properties make them particularly valuable for dealing with hay fever, skin irritation, and minor wounds. Examples include myrrh, sandalwood, and patchouli.

## Moving Forward

Although this is a brief overview of essential oil chemistry, it can give you insight into what type of action you might be able to expect from aromatherapy treatments that contain oils that are high in certain constituents. It would take an entire book to provide an in-depth analysis of the hundreds of essential oils available, especially because each oil has more than one hundred components. Further, when you combine essential oils with one another, a synergistic effect is produced; in short, the therapeutic action of each oil can be increased. In the next chapter, you'll learn how to put what you've learned so far into practice—and to do so safely.

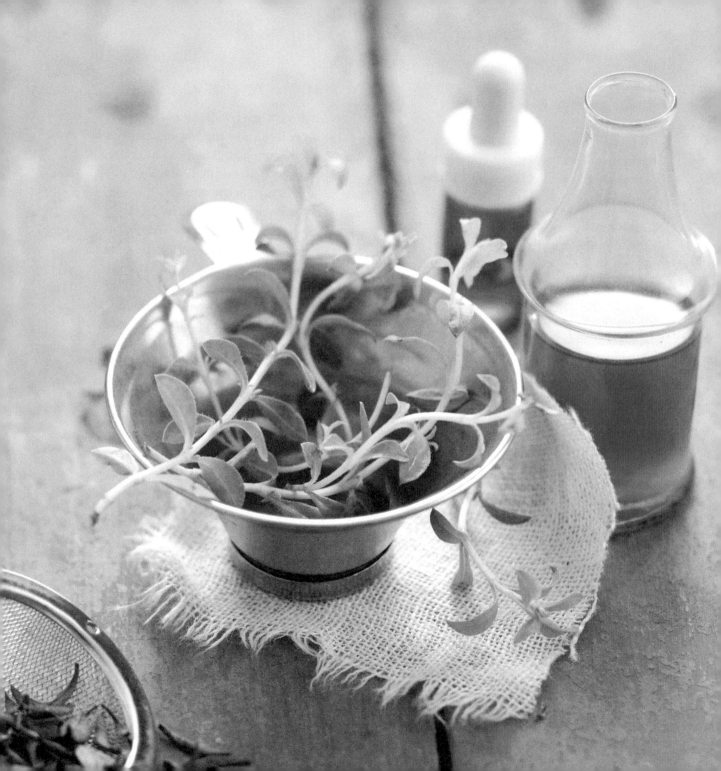

# THREE

# Rooted in Practice

As you'll soon discover, there are many ways to use aromatherapy as part of a natural lifestyle. You'll find full essential oil profiles in chapter 7, but before you jump in, it's important to learn how to choose good essential oils and carriers, mix basic aromatherapy recipes, and use them safely.

## Shopping for Oils

The moment you begin shopping for essential oils, you'll notice that there are many different brands to choose from. Not all essential oils are suitable for aromatherapy, but it is very easy to find quality products. Use the following tips to determine which brands are likely to be best.

**Avoid purchasing a product labeled** *fragrance oil.* Other watchwords to avoid include *perfume oil* and *identical oil.* These are not true essential oils.

**Know the difference between absolutes and pre-diluted oil.** Some very expensive absolutes, such as jasmine and rose, are available pre-diluted, meaning that they have been blended into a base oil. These are nice to have, and they cost much less than absolutes, but they cannot be substituted for absolutes, drop for drop, in aromatherapy recipes. If you purchase a pre-diluted oil, make sure the label contains the absolute's Latin name—for example, *Jasminum grandiflorum,* which is one of three jasmine varieties used to produce jasmine absolute.

**Talk with the vendor about their packing and shipping procedures before making a large-quantity purchase.** Most essential oils are packaged in dark-colored glass bottles, and some are packaged in metal containers. Some vendors who ship large quantities of essential oil cut costs and prevent breakage during shipping by packing their oils in plastic containers.

This is acceptable as long as the oils are transferred to the plastic containers just prior to shipping and as long as you transfer them into dark-colored glass bottles immediately upon receipt.

**Essential oil prices should vary widely within the same brand.** Very common oils like lemon and mandarin shouldn't cost much, but absolutes like jasmine and rose will have prices that may give you sticker shock. There should be plenty of other prices between the two extremes. If a vendor's oils all cost the same for the same amount, move on.

**Look for the Latin name on the label.** It's best to avoid essential oils with labels that fail to provide a Latin name for the plant from which the essential oil was obtained. There are many different varieties within species, and each variety has something different to offer.

**Read reviews and do your research.** A few companies sell their essential oils via multilevel marketing, a pyramid-type business practice in which individuals are compensated for the sales they generate and for sales made by the individuals they recruit. This is not necessarily a bad thing; in fact, you can get high-quality oils from most of these companies, along with some wonderful aromatherapy blends. Protect yourself by reading reviews and independently verifying any unusual claims being made before investing in the company's essential oils.

**There is no governing body that tests or regulates essential oils.** Most companies make statements concerning essential oil purity, and some take it a step further by mentioning that their products are "aromatherapy grade" or "therapeutic grade." Most sellers aren't trying to deceive you by providing this information, but it's best to conduct research about the product in question. After all, anyone can make marketing claims.

**If offered the option, consider choosing organic essential oil whenever possible.** As long as an organic oil stands up to your scrutiny and falls within your budget, go for it. While non-organic oils are certainly beneficial, organics are often superior. Of course, the choice is all yours.

Don't be afraid to buy essential oils online. Shopping online gives you access to more variety than most local stores are able to provide, and all major essential oil companies maintain strong online presences, complete with knowledgeable customer service representatives who are able to answer questions. Shopping online also gives you the ability to compare oils side by side with no pressure. As a bonus, many sources also offer tools for making aromatherapy products, as well as high-quality packaging in which to store balms, lotions, sprays, and other remedies.

## All About Carrier Oils

If you look in your kitchen cupboard, you'll probably find that you have at least one or two carrier oils on hand already. Carrier oils are vegetable oils that come from the fatty part of a plant; the majority come from nuts, seeds, and kernels.

You'll be using carrier oils to create aromatherapy treatments and to dilute essential oils before applying them to skin. There are several reasons to use carrier oils. First, they prevent strong essential oils from burning your skin. Second, they prevent the essential oils from evaporating quickly, which allows more molecules to be absorbed. Third, carrier oils can

### UNDERSTANDING ESSENTIAL OILS, HYDROSOLS, AND FLORAL WATERS

Essential oils are natural, volatile oils that have been extracted from the plants for which they are named. Why *essential*? The word is used not because these oils are necessary, but because they carry the very essence of a plant's unique fragrance.

Many essential oils are produced via steam, water, or water and steam distillation, and it is this process that produces hydrosols—the aromatic water that is left behind. In some cases, hydrosols are specially distilled for use in aromatherapy. Hydrosols smell fantastic, and they make wonderful additions to creams, lotions, and other skincare products. Hydrosols are also a good choice for creating natural perfumes. Rose, neroli, and lavender are among the most popular.

Unless you really love the smell and don't mind emptying your pocketbook, avoid floral waters, which are often mistaken for true hydrosols and are often made with a combination of water and essential oil, sometimes with chemicals added. You can easily make your own floral waters and essential oil spritzers to use as linen spray or to freshen air naturally while enjoying some mild aromatherapy benefits. All it takes is two or three drops of the oil of your choice, four ounces of distilled water, and an inexpensive spritzer bottle. Shake the blend before each use and enjoy. (You can find specific recipes for household sprays in chapter 6.)

offer health benefits of their own. They provide moisture, soothe irritation caused by conditions like psoriasis and eczema, and, in some cases, can help heal inflammation faster.

Each carrier oil has different properties and lends itself to a variety of uses. Here is a list of 22 of the most popular carrier oils:

- **Apricot kernel oil** good for massage blends, with a slippery, semi-oily feel.

- **Avocado oil** great for skin and hair, and a little goes a long way.

- **Black cumin seed oil** great for skin issues, indigestion, and immune system support.

- **Borage seed oil** high in omega-6 fatty acid; ideal for skin care.

- **Calendula oil** an infused oil made with calendula, not to be confused with calendula essential oil; excellent for use in first-aid treatments.

- **Cranberry seed oil** high in vitamin E; ideal for healing problem skin.

- **Evening primrose oil** a thin, lightweight oil that absorbs quickly; ideal for eczema.

- **Fractionated coconut oil** not to be confused with coconut oil, this lightweight option absorbs quickly and is a good choice for massage blends.

- **Grapeseed oil** an all-purpose carrier oil with a thin feel; can leave a sheen behind.

- **Hazelnut oil** lightweight, with a sweet, nutty smell; good for all-around use.

- **Hemp seed oil** great for healthy skin, hair, and nails; supports the immune system.

- **Jojoba oil** a natural anti-inflammatory; very good for problem skin.

- **Kukui nut oil** lightweight, slippery, and nourishing; ideal for eczema and psoriasis, and good for aging skin.

- **Macadamia nut** a rich, thick oil that leaves a film behind; very good for mixing with other carrier oils to create massage blends.

- **Meadowfoam seed oil** high in vitamin E, and highly shelf-stable; excellent for anti-aging treatments.

- **Olive oil** heavy-textured, inexpensive, and good in a pinch, when other carrier oils aren't available.

- **Pomegranate seed oil** high in antioxidants, with anti-inflammatory properties; good for skin irritation.

- **Rosehip oil** expensive, but excellent for aging or irritated skin.

- **Sea buckthorn berry oil** a blend of fruit pulp and seed oil; excellent for treating aging skin; has a bright orange color that can cause staining when used at high dilutions.

- **Sesame seed oil** an excellent all-purpose oil, but best for blending with lighter carriers as it has a strong sesame smell.

- **Sunflower oil** an affordable all-purpose carrier oil with a sweet, almost floral aroma; absorbs well.

- **Sweet almond oil** a medium-viscosity carrier that's good for all-purpose use; leaves behind a hint of oil on most skin types.

## Items to Have on Hand: Essential and Nice to Have

Here are some items to have on hand before you begin to craft aromatherapy recipes. You'll find some of these at your favorite kitchen store, and others are available for sale from companies that offer aromatherapy supplies. You may find items like dark-colored glass bottles at your local health food store, but you're likely to enjoy better prices by shopping for them online.

### ESSENTIALS

**Dark glass containers** These are essential for storing blends long term, because exposure to light shortens shelf life. There are many sizes and shapes available, ranging from glass bottles with misting spray tops or trigger spray tops to salve and cosmetics containers. Clear glass containers—even sanitized jam jars—will do in

a pinch, as long as you keep your remedies in a dark place.

**Glass or metal bowls** It's a good idea to get bowls in different sizes and to keep them separate from those used for food prep. Strong oils can damage plastic bowls and utensils; while they will do in a pinch, they're far from ideal. Whichever you choose, be sure to wash them well with soap and water after each use.

**Labels** These are a must for marking your blends. You can buy special labels that correspond with the containers you choose, or you can make your own with something as simple as masking tape.

**Liquid measuring cups** Get at least one liquid measuring cup to use for carrier oils. Most of the remedies in this book make eight ounces or less, so a one-cup measure might serve your purposes perfectly for now.

**Mini funnels** These are essential for filling bottles with narrow mouths. The typical size is 1½-inches wide at the top and ¼-inch wide at the bottom.

**Travel-size containers** If you plan to bring remedies along in a carry-on bag, travel-size containers are essential. They're available in glass or plastic; although plastic isn't ideal, it's okay for storing blends you plan to use within a week or two. You can justify the cost of glass ones by mixing up larger batches of

# OTHER INGREDIENTS TO HAVE ON HAND

Many recipes in this book call for some ingredients you may need in addition to essential oils and the carrier oils of your choice. This is by no means an exhaustive list, but it will help you stock up before getting started. When shopping, be sure to check expiration dates if applicable, and buy only what you need. Some items, such as beeswax, don't come with expiration dates, making it easy to save some money by purchasing in bulk.

- **Creams and waxes.** Beeswax, shea butter, cocoa butter, and virgin coconut oil make thick, creamy lotions, salves, and more.

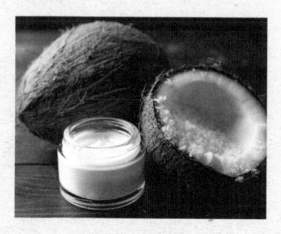

- **Dry ingredients.** Basics like baking soda, sugar, milk powder, and sea salt extend your repertoire, allowing you to make scented foot and body powders, bath salts, body scrubs, smelling salts, and other items. Diatomaceous earth comes in handy too for several recipes.

- **Liquids.** Vinegar, hydrogen peroxide, and alcohol-free witch hazel lend themselves to a variety of uses. Foot soaks, toners, and first-aid treatments are some of the recipes that call for these ingredients.

- **Natural body supplies.** Unscented all-natural body supplies such as shampoo, conditioner, and body wash offer convenience, allowing you to add essential oils that suit your needs. Liquid or bar castile soap is another staple to have on hand, particularly if you want to try your hand at formulating complicated body care recipes from scratch.

It's often fine to substitute similar ingredients for one another. For example, if a recipe calls for cocoa butter and you only have shea butter, feel free to use it.

your favorite portable remedies and then refilling your travel-size ones for continuous use on the go.

## NICE TO HAVE

**Essential oil dispensing syringe**  This is a good tool to have for making blends when recipes use increments marked in milliliters (ml) rather than drops. They are typically available in 1-ml increments. Medical syringes such as those found at drugstores will work too; just make sure that measurements are marked in milliliters.

**Glass droppers or disposable pipettes**
Droppers let you easily measure essential oils and other ingredients accurately. If you don't get droppers or pipettes, make sure that all of your essential oil bottles are fitted with orifice reducers, which are small discs that dispense one drop of liquid at a time.

**Glass roller bottles**  Rollers make using homemade lip balms, perfumes, and portable aromatherapy remedies more convenient.

**Massage chair or table**  If you really want to reap the rewards of aromatherapy, learn alongside a partner and use your blends in soothing massages. It's true that you can sit or lie anywhere to receive a massage, but massage chairs and tables make muscle groups

accessible, and they are much more comfortable for both parties.

**Metal measuring spoons**  Metal measuring spoons help you ensure accuracy when creating blends. Plastic will do in a pinch because you won't be using these for straight essential oils in most cases.

**Stirring utensils**  Special stirring utensils such as glass rods are nice to have, but not necessary. Although some recipes benefit from an electric hand mixer, a fork or whisk works nicely for most things; even a chopstick will do in a pinch.

# Application Methods and Supplies

Simple supplies, including a few items you may already have on hand, can enhance your enjoyment of aromatherapy and help you treat ailments efficiently. As you'll discover when you begin shopping for supplies, there are many wonderful things to choose from. Here are a few basics.

## AROMATIC

Inhalation of essential oils can be made easier with a few items. For starters, diffusers are essential to aromatherapy. It's true there are many pricey models out there that do a wonderful job of sending an aromatic mist into the air, but it's also true that simple terra-cotta discs, porous stones, and old-fashioned candle-powered diffusers can do the trick. My go-to diffuser is a very simple battery-operated model that I can take from place to place. It even comes along in the car!

Aromatherapy inhalers are also nice to have, offering an easy solution for inhaling essential oils and blends anywhere. There are a few different varieties available, mostly online.

Another option is aromatherapy jewelry, including pendants, bracelets, and earrings. Wearing aromatherapy jewelry lets you diffuse your desired scent right inside your personal space whenever you like. There are many different styles available for men and women, ranging from simple blown glass designs to intricate lockets.

### TOPICAL

Some topical applications don't require any special equipment; the blend is simply rubbed into the skin. In other cases, hot or cold application is recommended. There is a variety of ways to create hot and cold compresses that make aromatherapy treatments more effective. Simple ice packs and heating pads are excellent.

Reusable bags made with fabric and rice or buckwheat hulls can be stored in the freezer for use in cold therapy, or microwaved for a short time for use as a hot compress. Even simple folded cloths dipped in hot or iced water can be used to make compresses.

### INGESTION

None of the recipes in this book instruct you to consume essential oil. If you are interested in this method, you'll need to seek the help of an experienced aromatherapist. Vegetable caplets are an essential tool for ingestion, and an experienced aromatherapist will be able to supply what you need.

## Using Essential Oils Safely

Essential oils are powerful substances. Although they're all-natural, it's very important to follow these simple safety guidelines. If you suffer from a medical condition such as epilepsy, diabetes, or cancer, check to ensure that the essential oils you're considering don't come with specific health warnings related to your condition. Also, if you are allergic to certain plants or foods such as nuts, avoid essential oils or carrier oils made with them.

## ESSENTIAL OILS TO AVOID

The following oils are highly toxic, extremely irritating to skin or lungs, or even lethal if ingested. Some of these essential oils are used in perfumery, and some are described as safe by certain resources. It's always best to be safe and to avoid the following essential oils despite reports of their potential benefits.

- **Bitter almond** toxic; contains cyanide; small quantities can be lethal

- **Boldo leaf** toxic; can produce convulsions

- **Horseradish** caustic; can cause severe pain and inflammation

- **Mugwort** toxic; can cause miscarriage; neurotoxin

- **Mustard** caustic; burns skin; causes respiratory distress

- **Pennyroyal** toxic; causes liver damage; causes lung damage; can cause death if ingested

- **Rue** toxic; irritates lungs and mucous membranes; neurotoxin; can burn skin

- **Sassafras** carcinogenic; small quantities can be lethal

- **Savin** toxic; small quantities can be lethal

- **Tansy** toxic; can produce convulsions; can cause uterine bleeding; small quantities can be lethal (Note: This is not the same oil as blue tansy.)

- **Thuja** toxic; can cause severe gastro-intestinal distress; can cause convulsions; neurotoxin

- **Wintergreen** extremely toxic; even tiny quantities can be lethal

- **Wormseed** explosive; can explode when heated or combined with an acid; toxic to liver and kidneys; small quantities can be lethal; can cause deafness and vision loss

- **Wormwood** toxic; can cause addiction and brain damage; neurotoxin

## USING ESSENTIAL OILS WHILE PREGNANT

Many essential oils are emmenagogues, meaning that they promote menstruation. While those oils can be useful for treating painful periods and PMS, they should be avoided during pregnancy. Note that some emmenagogues, particularly jasmine and clary sage, are also parturient, meaning that they can assist with labor and delivery. If you'd like to use essential oils in the delivery room, ensure that you do so with the help of an experienced aromatherapist, doula, or midwife.

Many of the recipes used in this book call for one or a combination of the oils listed next, so keep substitution oils on hand. For pregnant people, lavender and spearmint are two of the best substitution oils, and mix well in most recipes.

If you are pregnant and considering a specific oil, conduct some research beforehand to ensure that it is safe.

- Angelica
- Anise (also known as aniseed)
- Bay laurel
- Caraway seed
- Carrot seed
- Catnip
- Cedarwood
- Chamomile (German and Roman)
- Cinnamon leaf
- Clary sage
- Copaiba
- Davana
- Elemi
- Eucalyptus
- Fennel seed
- Frankincense
- Ginger
- Hops flower
- Hyssop
- Jasmine
- Juniper
- Marjoram
- Lavandin
- Myrrh
- Myrtle
- Oregano
- Peppermint
- Ravintsara
- Rose
- Rosemary
- Spanish sage
- Tagetes
- Vitex berry

## USING OILS WITH CARE

It's important to be careful with all essential oils, but some do come with particular warnings. Keep essential oils—even those safe for use with small children—out of reach of youngsters. Also, be sure to check for contraindications before using any essential oil for the first time.

When an essential oil has the potential to cause sensitive skin, dilute it with at least twice as much carrier oil. In other words, use at least two drops of carrier oil for every one drop of essential oil. Also, use it with great care on children under 12 as well as with those who are frail, elderly, wheelchair-bound, or bedridden. It's also a good idea to avoid these essential oils during pregnancy, as skin can be extra-sensitive during this special time.

If you are breastfeeding or taking care of an infant, you'll need to take extra precautions when using essential oils that can cause sensitive skin, as they are absorbed by your body and could be unintentionally passed on to a vulnerable baby.

Be aware that different resources provide contradictory information, and err on the side of safety rather than taking chances.

- **Allspice** may cause sensitive skin

- **Anise** also known as aniseed; avoid if diagnosed with any form of cancer

- **Basil** avoid if diagnosed with any form of cancer; may cause sensitive skin

- **Bay** avoid if diagnosed with any form of cancer; may cause sensitive skin

- **Benzoin** may cause sensitive skin; avoid if driving or operating machinery

- **Bergamot** avoid if diagnosed with melanoma or skin cancer; may cause sensitive skin

- **Birch** may cause sensitive skin

- **Black pepper** may cause sensitive skin

- **Camphor** avoid if diagnosed with epilepsy

- **Carnation** avoid if driving or operating machinery

- **Cassia** may cause sensitive skin

- **Cedarwood** may cause sensitive skin

- **Chamomile (German and Roman)** avoid if driving or operating machinery

- **Cinnamon** avoid both cinnamon leaf and cinnamon bark if diagnosed with any form of cancer; may cause sensitive skin

- **Citronella** avoid if diagnosed with estrogen-dependent cancer; may cause sensitive skin

- **Clove bud** avoid if diagnosed with any form of cancer; may cause sensitive skin

- **Costus** may cause sensitive skin

- **Cumin** may cause sensitive skin

- **Elecampane** may cause sensitive skin

- **Eucalyptus** avoid all species if diagnosed with estrogen-dependent cancer; *Eucalyptus globulus* may cause sensitive skin

- **Fennel seed** avoid if diagnosed with any form of cancer; may cause sensitive skin

- **Fir needle** may cause sensitive skin

- **Geranium** avoid if driving or operating machinery

- **Ginger** may cause sensitive skin

- **Grapefruit** avoid if diagnosed with melanoma or skin cancer

## PHOTOTOXIC OILS AND SUN SENSITIVITY

Essential oils may be completely natural, but some, including many citrus varieties, can cause a side effect known as phototoxicity. When exposed to direct sunlight, they can increase the skin's susceptibility to sunburn. You can use oils such as lemon, lime, and grapefruit on days that you plan to spend time in the sun, as long as you don't apply them to areas that will be directly exposed to sunlight. Lotions, lip balms, and perfumes are examples of products that stay put and can cause a problem with phototoxicity. Soaps, body washes, shampoos, and other treatments that will be rinsed off do not present a risk, since they do not remain on your skin.

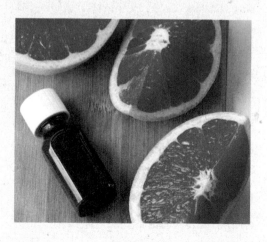

- **Helichrysum** may cause sensitive skin
- **Ho leaf** avoid if diagnosed with any form of cancer
- **Hops** avoid if driving or operating machinery
- **Hyacinth** avoid if driving or operating machinery
- **Hyssop** avoid if diagnosed with epilepsy; avoid if diagnosed with high blood pressure
- **Juniper** may cause sensitive skin
- **Laurel** avoid if diagnosed with any form of cancer
- **Lavender** avoid if driving or operating machinery
- **Lemon verbena** may cause sensitive skin
- **Lemon** avoid if diagnosed with melanoma or skin cancer; may cause sensitive skin
- **Lemongrass** avoid if diagnosed with estrogen-dependent cancer; may cause sensitive skin
- **Lime** avoid if diagnosed with melanoma or skin cancer
- **Linden blossom** avoid if driving or operating machinery
- **Mace** avoid if driving or operating machinery

- **Mandarin**  avoid if diagnosed with melanoma or skin cancer

- **Marjoram**  avoid if driving or operating machinery

- **Melissa**  may cause sensitive skin

- **Neroli**  avoid if driving or operating machinery

- **Nutmeg**  avoid if diagnosed with any form of cancer; may cause sensitive skin; avoid if driving or operating machinery

- **Oak moss**  may cause sensitive skin

- **Oregano**  may cause sensitive skin

- **Ormenis flower**  avoid if driving or operating machinery

- **Parsley seed**  may cause sensitive skin

- **Peppermint**  avoid if diagnosed with heart problems; may cause sensitive skin

- **Petitgrain**  avoid if driving or operating machinery

- **Pine**  may cause sensitive skin

- **Rosemary**  avoid if diagnosed with epilepsy or high blood pressure

- **Sage**  avoid if diagnosed with epilepsy or high blood pressure

- **Sandalwood**  avoid if driving or operating machinery

- **Spike lavender**  avoid if diagnosed with epilepsy

- **Spikenard**  avoid if driving or operating machinery

- **Star anise**  avoid if diagnosed with estrogen-dependent cancer

- **Sweet orange**  avoid if diagnosed with melanoma or skin cancer; may cause sensitive skin

- **Tagetes**  may cause sensitive skin

- **Tangerine**  avoid if diagnosed with melanoma or skin cancer

- **Thyme**  may cause sensitive skin; avoid if diagnosed with high blood pressure

- **Valerian**  avoid if driving or operating machinery

- **Verbena**  avoid if diagnosed with estrogen-dependent cancer

- **Vetiver**  avoid if driving or operating machinery

- **Ylang-ylang**  avoid if driving or operating machinery

# FIVE COMMON MISTAKES
## WHEN PRACTICING AROMATHERAPY

Start reading about aromatherapy, and you'll find that there are quite a few strong statements and opinions floating around. These can make it tough to distinguish myth from fact. Here's a short list of some of the most common mistakes and challenges many people experience when incorporating essential oils into their lives.

1. **Believing that only certain oils are pure or therapeutic.** Labels can make it difficult to ascertain which essential oils are appropriate for aromatherapy use. Some companies use marketing language that makes it seem as if their brand is the only one that is safe and effective to use, while others choose not to. In reality, there are many wonderful companies that provide pure essential oils suitable for aromatherapy.

2. **Thinking that essential oils are natural, and they will never cause harm.** As stated in the previous safety section, there are essential oils that can cause a wide range of problems, including a few dangerous ones that can cause serious illness or death.

3. **Not diluting essential oils properly before use.** Almost all essential oils need to be diluted before use, especially when applied to anyone with a developing or compromised body. Some essential oils can be used neat (that is, without being diluted); however, it's best to err on the side of safety if you are uncertain.

4. **Believing that essential oil bottles marked "for external use only" should be avoided.** This is a warning that most essential oil companies place on their bottles out of concern for your safety. A few companies advise their customers to avoid products with these labels, but like claims about purity or grade, this is merely marketing language.

5. **Forgetting to look for the Latin name when shopping for essential oils.** Certain plant families like lavender, eucalyptus, and tea tree contain multiple species, and each has different properties. Verifying which essential oil you purchase helps ensure you are receiving the desired therapeutic action and keeps you safe.

## PATCH TEST

Because it's difficult to predict how a specific essential oil will affect your skin, it's best to conduct a patch test before use, even if you are not normally sensitive. Take extra care with patch testing whenever an essential oil is listed as having the potential to cause sensitive skin.

To conduct a patch test, combine one drop of the essential oil in question with one teaspoon of carrier oil. Apply a single drop of this blend to your inner elbow, and leave it alone for 24 hours. Do not wash the area during the test period unless irritation develops.

If, after the 24-hour test period passes, you have no sign of redness, itching, or swelling, then it should be safe for you to use the essential oil you're considering.

Because carrier oils can cause sensitive skin, too, it's best to perform a patch test using one drop of each new carrier oil before using it on larger areas of skin or combining it with essential oils for patch testing.

# Aromatherapy Intentions

When used correctly, aromatherapy supports good health and helps you deal with issues such as muscle pain, respiratory concerns, insomnia,

and much more. Choosing the right essential oils is a personal matter, whether you plan to enjoy their beautiful aromas in your home or office, or if you plan to use them for skin care, massage, or to treat common ailments.

Remember that essential oils are highly concentrated. While they provide many benefits, it's vital to follow safety guidelines. Doing so will protect you, your family, and even your pets from suffering sensitivity or illness.

It's true that some essential oils are safe for internal use, but only under the guidance of a trained aromatherapist or clinician who understands the safety implications associated with the essential oils that you are considering. Don't fall into the trap of believing that ingestion is the best way to take your essential oils; remember, inhalation and topical application are effective ways to deliver beneficial constituents to all of your body's sensitive systems, with far decreased risks of unpleasant or dangerous side effects.

Making and using aromatherapy products is an enjoyable process. In the coming chapters, you'll learn how to use aromatherapy for health and wellness, beauty, and around the house.

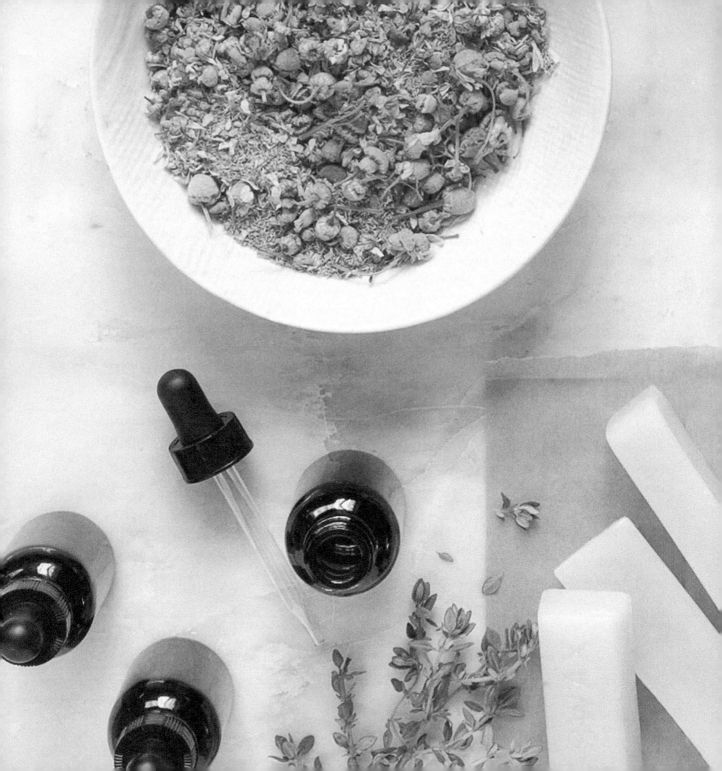

# FOUR

# Remedies for Health & Wellness

The essential oils used in aromatherapy are versatile and, with the power of many pounds of plant material packed into every drop, they provide effective healing for a wide range of common health problems. This chapter contains more than 250 fragrant remedies, offering you an extensive array of choices that put you in charge of your own health and wellness.

Remember to check each essential oil's profile in chapter 7 and use your best judgment when determining whether to treat an issue yourself or see the doctor; if you are in doubt, err on the side of safety and seek medical treatment before turning to aromatherapy.

Essential oils should be capped tightly and stored in a cool, dark place. Unless otherwise noted, any treatments you make with essential oils that are not used immediately should be treated the same way.

# ABSCESSES

Painful and hot to touch, abscesses can appear anywhere on the body. A small abscess generally responds well to aromatherapy, but seek medical attention if the abscess is larger than one centimeter across.

## Bergamot Compress

Makes 1 treatment

Bergamot essential oil is a potent antiseptic. Combined with Epsom salt and warm water, and then applied as a warm compress, it treats infection while reducing inflammation.

1 cup warm water
1 teaspoon Epsom salt
2 drops bergamot essential oil

1. In a large bowl, dissolve the Epsom salt in the warm water, and then add the essential oil.

2. Soak a folded washcloth in the solution, and then lay it on top of your abscess. Top the washcloth with a folded hand towel to catch any drips.

3. Leave the compress in place for 10 to 15 minutes. Repeat three to four times daily until the abscess is gone.

SUBSTITUTION TIP If you don't have bergamot essential oil, you can use lavender in its place.

## Four-Oil Abscess Salve

Makes 36 treatments

With lavender and chamomile to soothe inflammation, plus tea tree and thyme to stop infection, this blend is potent. The fractionated coconut oil provides additional antibacterial action.

24 drops fractionated coconut oil
4 drops thyme essential oil
3 drops tea tree essential oil
3 drops lavender essential oil
2 drops German or Roman chamomile essential oil

1. In a small bottle or jar, combine all the ingredients. Shake well to blend.

2. With a cotton swab, apply 1 drop of the blend to the abscess after using a compress or bathing. Reapply 4 to 6 times daily until the abscess is gone.

PREFERENCE TIP If you like the fragrance of this salve and have any left over, you can add a few drops to your diffuser or use the blend in a relaxing bath.

## Chamomile-Tea Tree Bath Salts

Makes 8 treatments

Chamomile and tea tree essential oils combine with Epsom salt to soothe inflammation and stop infection. This treatment is best for abscesses in hard-to-reach areas that are difficult to treat with salves or compresses.

2 tablespoons fractionated coconut oil
24 drops tea tree essential oil
16 drops Roman chamomile essential oil
4 cups Epsom salt

1. In a large bowl, combine the fractionated coconut oil and the essential oils. Add the Epsom salt and stir well to blend. Transfer the bath salts to a jar.

2. Draw a hot bath and add ½ cup of the bath salts. Soak in the bath for at least 15 minutes. Repeat once daily until the abscess is gone.

# ANXIOUSNESS

Whatever its cause, anxiousness is a disruptive emotion that makes life seem difficult. Aromatherapy helps by promoting feelings of peace and tranquility.

## Calming Temple Rub

Makes 150 treatments

Soothing and uplifting essential oils combine to produce a sense of calm confidence. This blend is ideal for carrying along in a bag or briefcase.

1 tablespoon sweet almond oil
10 drops lavender essential oil
10 drops rose geranium essential oil
10 drops sandalwood essential oil
4 drops ylang-ylang essential oil

1. In a small bottle, preferably with a roll-on applicator, combine all the ingredients. Shake well to blend.

2. With your fingertips or the roller, apply 1 drop to each temple and gently massage the area. Repeat as needed.

STORAGE  Keep in a convenient location if you plan to use it up within a few weeks; otherwise, keep in a cool, dark place for up to a year.

## Relaxing Lavender-Vetiver-Rose Bedtime Lotion

Makes 16 treatments

When anxious thoughts cause restlessness, this trio creates a soothing fragrance that helps you put your worries to bed so you can rest.

8 ounces unscented body lotion
40 drops lavender essential oil
40 drops vetiver essential oil
4 drops rose otto or rose absolute

1. In a large bowl, combine all the ingredients. Whisk to blend thoroughly, and then transfer the lotion to a jar or back to its original container.

2. Apply 1 tablespoon of lotion to your hands, arms, and shoulders as you are preparing for bed. Breathe deeply while relaxing. Repeat nightly as necessary.

STORAGE Keep this lotion in your nightstand if you plan to use it all within two weeks; otherwise, keep it in a glass bottle or jar in a cool, dark place.

SUBSTITUTION TIP You can use pre-diluted rose otto in this blend for a fraction of the cost. You'll need about 20 drops of the pre-diluted oil for each drop of the absolute.

## Yuzu-Ylang-Ylang Diffusion

Makes 10 treatments

This blend relies on yuzu and ylang-ylang to addresses two main components of anxiousness by uplifting the spirit and relieving stress.

24 drops yuzu essential oil
6 drops ylang-ylang essential oil

In a small bottle, combine the essential oils. Shake well to blend. Add 3 drops of the blend to your diffuser according to the manufacturer's instructions. Run the diffuser nearby and enjoy. Repeat as needed each day.

PREFERENCE TIP If you prefer florals, add another 1 or 2 drops of ylang-ylang; for a stronger citrus scent, add 4 to 6 more drops of yuzu.

# AROUSAL

Set the scene for romance with aromatherapy blends that enhance arousal by appealing to the senses and stimulating passion. These wonderful scents also address stress, making it much easier to focus on your partner.

## Sensual Massage Oil

Makes about 4 ounces

This intoxicating blend includes ginger and ylang-ylang to promote feelings of intense happiness and heighten attraction. Sandalwood and patchouli promote euphoria, and mandarin provides a yummy citrus note.

4 ounces sweet almond oil
16 drops sandalwood essential oil
6 drops mandarin essential oil
4 drops patchouli essential oil
2 drops ginger essential oil
2 drops ylang-ylang essential oil

1. In a bottle or jar, combine all the ingredients. Shake well to blend.

2. After bathing or showering, pat yourself dry and apply 1 teaspoon of the blend to your shoulders, neck, and upper arms, and massage in. Add a little more to your legs and other areas if you like.

## Jasmine Linen Spray

*Makes 8 ounces*

Jasmine offers a soothing, sensual scent that promotes feelings of love, peace, and emotional warmth. Use this spray to give your bedroom's curtains, carpet, and linens a lingering scent. It's nice as a hair and body spritz, too.

8 ounces distilled water
4 drops jasmine absolute

1. In a bottle with a fine-mist spray top, combine the ingredients. Shake well to blend, and then shake again before each use.

2. Spray liberally on linens, carpets, and curtains.

SUBSTITUTION TIP Jasmine absolute is costly, so many companies offer this oil pre-diluted. If you use pre-diluted jasmine in this recipe, use 10 to 20 drops for each drop of jasmine absolute.

## Rose-Davana Perfume

*Makes 150 treatments*

Exotic davana and rose come together with a touch of tangerine to create a flirty, feminine scent. Davana is unique from all other essential oils in that it smells different on everyone. Wear this on your pulse points for a unique, alluring fragrance.

1 tablespoon sweet almond oil
8 drops rose otto or rose absolute
8 drops mandarin essential oil
2 drops davana essential oil

1. In a small bottle, preferably with a roll-on applicator, combine all the ingredients. Shake well to blend.

2. With your fingertips or the roller, apply 1 drop to the pulse point behind each ear, and gently massage the area. If a stronger personal fragrance is desired, apply 1 drop to each wrist, your throat, or your inner elbows.

STORAGE Keep in a convenient location if you plan to use it up within a few weeks; otherwise, keep in a cool, dark place for up to a year.

# ARTHRITIS

Inflammation and joint stiffness make arthritis a painful, debilitating ailment. Aromatherapy can bring relief in many mild to moderate cases and can be used alongside stronger medicines when symptoms are severe.

## Soothing Marjoram Balm

Makes 1 ounce

Marjoram offers warm, soothing relief, and black cumin seed oil helps with inflammation. Marjoram enhances relaxation, so avoid driving until you know how your body reacts.

**1 ounce black cumin seed essential oil**
**3 drops marjoram essential oil**

1. In a bottle or jar, combine the ingredients. Shake well to blend.

2. With your fingertips, apply 1 drop of the blend to each affected area, and gently massage the area. Repeat every 2 to 3 hours as needed.

## Eucalyptus Radiata Spray

Makes about 4 ounces

*Eucalyptus radiata* oil is a strong anti-inflammatory oil that is safe for seniors. You can combine this spray with a warm or cold compress to intensify the feeling of relief.

1 ounce **aloe vera gel**
1 ounce **grapeseed oil**
1 ounce **vitamin E oil**
1 ounce **distilled water**
40 drops *Eucalyptus radiata* **essential oil**

1. In a bottle with a fine-mist spray top, combine all the ingredients. Shake well to blend, and then shake again before each use.

2. Apply 1 spritz to each affected joint, and massage the area if desired. Use as often as needed.

SUBSTITUTION TIP You can replace the *Eucalyptus radiata* with *Eucalyptus globulus* or lemon eucalyptus essential oil; however, reduce the amount to 30 drops.

STORAGE If you like, you can keep this spray in the refrigerator for an intense cooling sensation upon application; otherwise, keep in a cool, dark place.

## Synergistic Arthritis Massage Oil

Makes about 4 ounces

Peppermint, black pepper, Roman chamomile, and lavender essential oils offer anesthetic, analgesic, and anti-inflammatory properties that ease the pain and inflammation that accompany arthritis.

4 ounces **hemp seed oil**
40 drops **peppermint essential oil**
40 drops **Roman chamomile essential oil**
10 drops **black pepper essential oil**
10 drops **lavender essential oil**

1. In a bottle or jar, combine all the ingredients. Shake well to blend.

2. Apply 1 drop of the blend to small joints such as fingers; apply a dime-size amount to larger joints such as knees, ankles, or elbows, and massage the area. Repeat as needed.

SUBSTITUTION TIP If you're missing the Roman chamomile, black pepper, and/or lavender essential oils, use more peppermint; it can be an effective joint pain remedy on its own in this recipe.

# ASTHMA

With wheezing and shortness of breath that can lead to feelings of panic, asthma sufferers experience intense physical and emotional discomfort. Aromatherapy treatments help address both issues. Keep in mind that asthma is a serious illness, so be sure to let your doctor know that you're using aromatherapy alongside prescribed treatments.

## Cajuput-Bergamot Diffusion

Makes 1 treatment

Cajuput is a strong decongestant that promotes easy breathing, and bergamot addresses fear and stress. Both essential oils offer antispasmodic properties to help keep the muscles around the airway relaxed.

**2 drops bergamot essential oil**
**1 drop cajuput essential oil**

1. Add the essential oils to your diffuser according to the manufacturer's instructions.
2. Run the diffuser nearby. Repeat as needed.

## Relaxing Clary Sage-Lavender Chest Rub

Makes about 2 ounces

Clary sage and lavender offer anti-inflammatory, antispasmodic, and sedative properties that provide relief while offering a potent calming effect. Avoid driving or attempting tasks that require concentration after use.

2 ounces coconut oil, melted
30 drops lavender essential oil
15 drops clary sage essential oil

1. In a medium bowl, combine all the ingredients. Whisk to blend thoroughly, and then transfer the rub to a small jar.

2. Every 5 minutes or so, stir with a small spatula. Allow it to cool completely before capping.

3. With your fingertips, apply ½ teaspoon of salve to your chest, and massage the area. Repeat as needed, up to three times daily.

## Synergistic Asthma Inhaler

Makes 1 reusable inhaler

Refreshing pine, eucalyptus, tea tree, thyme, frankincense, and myrrh essential oils combine to help you expel mucus and breathe easier, while relaxing the muscles surrounding the airway.

6 drops eucalyptus essential oil
6 drops pine essential oil
6 drops tea tree essential oil
4 drops frankincense essential oil
4 drops myrrh essential oil
4 drops thyme essential oil

1. In a small bottle, combine all the ingredients. Shake well to blend.

2. Apply the blend to the cotton wick of the aromatherapy inhaler.

3. Hold the inhaler beneath your nose, and inhale slowly through both nostrils to a count of five. Hold your breath for another count of five, and then exhale slowly. Repeat as needed to prevent and soothe symptoms.

SUBSTITUTION TIP If you don't have an inhaler, you can transfer the blend to a small, dark glass bottle and inhale directly from the bottle or place 3 drops of the blend in your diffuser.

# ATHLETE'S FOOT

Intense itching and scaly skin on your feet are signs you've got athlete's foot. This fungal infection responds very well to aromatherapy treatments, especially when you address symptoms as soon as you notice them.

## Clove Bud Spray

Makes about 4 ounces

Clove bud is a potent antifungal that makes short work of athlete's foot. You can use this spicy-smelling spray on floors and shoes, too.

**4 ounces distilled water**
**40 drops clove bud essential oil**

1. In a bottle with a fine-mist spray top, combine the ingredients. Shake well to blend, and then shake again before each use.

2. Apply 1 spritz to each affected area once or twice daily. Continue treatments for 1 week after symptoms subside. Be sure to sanitize shoes and areas where you've walked barefoot.

## May Chang Foot Powder

Makes about 8 ounces

May Chang essential oil offers a fantastic fruity-spicy fragrance with strong lemon tones, and it also happens to be a strong antifungal agent. This powder is excellent for feet and shoes alike.

½ cup non-GMO cornstarch
½ cup baking soda
40 drops May Chang essential oil

1. In a medium bowl, combine all the ingredients. Whisk to blend thoroughly.

2. Sift the blend into a second bowl to remove any lumps, and then transfer the powder to a glass or metal sugar shaker.

3. Apply a single shake of powder to each foot. Be sure to get between the toes. Repeat once or twice daily to treat or prevent athlete's foot.

## Tea Tree Neat Treatment

Makes 1 treatment

Tea tree is one of a few essential oils that can be applied neat, and it soothes itching while killing fungi. Be sure to conduct a patch test before using this neat treatment. If you have sensitive skin, apply a layer of carrier oil to each affected area before applying the tea tree.

1 drop tea tree essential oil

1. Wash and dry your feet. With a cotton swab, apply a drop of tea tree oil to each affected area.

2. Repeat once or twice daily, continuing treatment for 3 to 4 days after symptoms disappear.

# BACKACHE

Strain, pregnancy, and long hours spent in a seated position are some of the things that can cause a backache. Aromatherapy provides prompt relief, especially if someone is available to give you a massage.

## Cedarwood Massage Oil

Makes about 1 ounce

Cedarwood essential oil offers an anti-spasmodic property that helps muscle fibers relax. It is also a mild sedative that makes for a pleasant massage.

**1 ounce sweet almond oil**
**20 drops cedarwood essential oil**

1. In a small bottle or jar, combine the ingredients. Shake well to blend.

2. With your fingertips, apply ½ teaspoon of the blend to the achy portion of your back, and massage the area, using light pressure. Repeat as needed.

## Lavender-Benzoin Bath Salts

Makes 8 treatments

Benzoin and lavender combine with Epsom salt to offer quick pain relief. This blend is strongly sedative, so it's best for times when you don't need to drive or focus on important tasks.

1 tablespoon fractionated coconut oil
16 drops benzoin essential oil
16 drops lavender essential oil
4 cups Epsom salt

1. In a large bowl, combine the essential oils and the fractionated coconut oil. Add the Epsom salt and stir well to blend. Transfer the bath salts to a jar.

2. Draw a hot bath and dissolve ½ cup of bath salts in the water. Soak in the bath for at least 15 minutes. Repeat as needed.

## Cinnamon Leaf-Ginger Salve

Makes about 4 ounces

Spicy cinnamon leaf and ginger offer analgesic and antispasmodic properties that ease discomfort while providing penetrating warmth. Benzoin increases pain relief while lending a note of vanilla fragrance to the blend.

¼ cup grapeseed oil
¼ cup sweet almond oil
2 tablespoons beeswax, melted
½ tablespoon vitamin E oil
10 drops ginger essential oil
5 drops cinnamon leaf essential oil
4 drops benzoin essential oil

1. In a medium bowl, combine all the ingredients. Stir well to blend, and then transfer the mixture to a wide-mouth jar and allow it to cool for 2 hours.

2. Apply ½ teaspoon of the blend to the achy portion of your back, and massage the area. Use a little more or less as needed. Repeat two to three times daily while discomfort persists.

# BLISTERS

Aromatherapy treatments are ideal for blisters caused by friction, but if you've been burned or have a large, painful blister, you should see your doctor before using essential oils.

## Lavender Neat Treatment

Makes 1 treatment

Lavender is one of a few essential oils that can be applied neat. Its analgesic and antiseptic properties combine to bring healing and quick relief from pain. Be sure to conduct a patch test before using this neat treatment.

**1 drop lavender essential oil**

1. Wash the affected area, and then pat it dry.

2. Apply the lavender essential oil by dripping it directly onto the blister from the bottle, being careful not to touch the bottle to the blister.

3. Repeat the treatment every 3 to 4 hours or as needed.

## Roman Chamomile-Tea Tree Balm

Makes 1 tablespoon

Roman chamomile and tea tree combine to offer quick pain relief and protection from infection. If your blister has popped, this is a good remedy to apply.

1 tablespoon fractionated coconut oil
10 drops Roman chamomile essential oil
10 drops tea tree essential oil

1. In a small bottle, combine all the ingredients. Shake well to blend.

2. Apply the blend by dripping 1 to 2 drops directly onto the blister, being careful not to touch the bottle to the blister.

3. Repeat the treatment every 3 to 4 hours or as needed.

## Myrrh-Helichrysum Compress

Makes 1 treatment

Myrrh and helichrysum combine with cold water to bring rapid pain relief while providing protection from infection.

½ cup distilled water
2 ice cubes
1 drop helichrysum essential oil
1 drop myrrh essential oil

1. In a small bowl, pour the distilled water over the ice cubes, and then add the essential oils.

2. Soak a folded washcloth in the solution, and then place it on the blister. Top the washcloth with a folded hand towel to catch any drips.

3. Leave the compress in place for 15 minutes. Allow your skin to air-dry after removal, and repeat as needed.

PREFERENCE TIP If you want to treat your blistered foot to a healing footbath instead, make this treatment in a shallow basin large enough to accommodate your foot. Double or triple the ingredients as needed. Soak your foot for 15 minutes, and then allow it to air-dry.

# BLOATING

Overeating, drinking carbonated beverages, and eating too quickly are just a few of the things that lead to uncomfortable bloating. These gentle treatments help you feel like yourself again, with no unpleasant side effects.

## Ginger-Black Pepper Digestive Massage

Makes 1 treatment

If overindulging on rich food is the cause of your bloating, try this quick treatment. Ginger and black pepper help move things along by increasing circulation and speeding digestion.

**1 tablespoon carrier oil**
**3 drops black pepper essential oil**
**1 drop ginger essential oil**

1.  In a small bowl, combine all the ingredients. Stir well to blend.

2.  Apply the entire blend to your abdomen, and massage the area, using clockwise motions. Spend 15 minutes lying on your left side, if possible, to help the gas pass from your system more quickly.

## Minty Orange-Chamomile Lotion

Makes about 4 ounces

Peppermint, sweet orange, and chamomile essential oils combine with unscented body lotion to enhance digestion and help prevent uncomfortable bloating.

4 ounces unscented body lotion
15 drops Roman or German chamomile essential oil
15 drops sweet orange essential oil
10 drops peppermint essential oil

1. In a medium bowl, combine all the ingredients. Whisk to blend thoroughly, and then transfer the lotion to a bottle or jar.

2. Apply 1 teaspoon of the lotion to your abdomen before eating a meal that's likely to trigger indigestion. Repeat as needed.

STORAGE Keep this lotion in a convenient location if you plan to use it all within two weeks; otherwise, keep it in a glass bottle or jar in a cool, dark place.

## Cinnamon Leaf-Fennel Seed Balm

Makes about 2 ounces

Fennel seed and cinnamon leaf increase circulation and enhance digestion, helping get your bloated belly back down to size.

1 tablespoon coconut oil, melted
1 tablespoon hemp oil
1 tablespoon shea butter
1 tablespoon sweet almond oil
16 drops fennel seed essential oil
12 drops cinnamon leaf essential oil

1. In a medium bowl, combine all the ingredients. Whisk to blend thoroughly, and then transfer the balm to a small jar.

2. Apply 1 teaspoon of the balm to your abdomen, and massage the area, using firm clockwise strokes. Repeat as often as needed.

# BODY ODOR

Body odor doesn't have to be a fact of life even if you're avoiding commercial deodorants with harmful ingredients. Try these natural solutions for smelling fresh and clean, 24/7.

## Rosewood Deodorant

Makes about 4 ounces

Fragrant rosewood combined with coconut oil and nourishing shea butter prevent fungal growth and stop odor. This deodorant offers gender-neutral appeal, thanks to its soft, woody aroma.

1 ounce coconut oil, melted
1 tablespoon arrowroot powder
1 tablespoon beeswax, melted
1 tablespoon food-grade diatomaceous earth
1 tablespoon shea butter
1 tablespoon sweet almond oil
25 drops rosewood essential oil
10 drops vitamin E oil

1. In a large bowl, combine all the ingredients. Whisk to blend thoroughly.

2. Pour the blend into a jar and allow it to cool completely before capping.

3. With your fingertips, apply a pea-size amount of the blend to each armpit, and massage the deodorant in, using light strokes, until absorbed. Repeat once or twice daily as needed.

# Lavender Body Powder

Makes about 8 ounces

Lavender offers antibacterial and antifungal properties, making it a good choice for dealing with body odor. If you prefer a masculine scent, replace the lavender with lemon eucalyptus.

2 ounces baking soda
40 drops lavender essential oil
4 ounces non-GMO cornstarch
2 ounces rice flour
1 teaspoon uncooked rice
   (optional, for humidity control)

1. In a large measuring cup, combine the baking soda and essential oil. Stir well to combine.

2. Sift the mixture into a large bowl, and then add the cornstarch and rice flour. Whisk to blend thoroughly. If you live in a humid climate, add the rice to keep the powder from clumping, and mix in well. Transfer the powder to a glass or metal sugar shaker.

3. Sprinkle about ½ teaspoon of powder onto the palm of your hand, and then apply to underarms and other body parts.

# Minty Rosemary-Patchouli Body Spray

Makes about 8 ounces

Peppermint, rosemary, and patchouli combine to keep you smelling fresh and clean. As an added benefit, this spray is an all-natural insect repellent.

7 ounces distilled water
1 ounce witch hazel
12 drops patchouli essential oil
10 drops peppermint essential oil
5 drops rosemary essential oil

1. In a bottle with a fine-mist spray top, combine all the ingredients. Shake well to blend, and then shake again before each use.

2. Apply 1 spritz to each area of your body you'd like to address.

# BOILS

Red, painful, and inflamed, boils often develop along the hairline, on the buttocks, in the groin area, or under the arms. If a boil worsens, enlarges, or begins to develop red streaks, seek medical attention and save aromatherapy treatment for another time.

## Synergistic Hot Compress

Makes 1 treatment

Antibacterial juniper berry, chamomile, tea tree, and lavender oils combine to create a strong disinfectant that kills germs while putting a stop to pain and swelling. Hot water opens the pores to speed delivery.

½ cup hot water
2 drops lavender essential oil
2 drops tea tree essential oil
1 drop juniper berry essential oil
1 drop Roman or German chamomile
   essential oil

1. In a medium bowl, combine all the ingredients.

2. Soak a folded washcloth in the blend and apply it to the boil. Top the washcloth with a folded hand towel to catch any drips.

3. Leave the compress in place for 15 minutes. Repeat two to three times daily until the boil is gone.

## Tea Tree Steam Treatment

Makes 1 treatment

Tea tree and steam from a hot towel work together to kill bacteria and speed healing. Be sure that the water you use is steaming, but not so hot that it scalds your skin.

**1 drop tea tree essential oil**
**1 cup steaming hot water**

1. With a cotton swab, apply the tea tree essential oil to the boil.

2. Dip a folded washcloth into the hot water and wring it out. Gently place the cloth over the boil, and without applying pressure, keep it in place until the heat dissipates.

3. Repeat two to three times daily until the boil is gone.

## Chamomile-Helichrysum Gel

Makes 1 ounce

Comforting chamomile and helichrysum combine with aloe vera gel to soothe and heal painful boils. You can use this blend on boils that have drained, as well as on those that are still developing.

**1 ounce aloe vera gel**
**6 drops German or Roman chamomile essential oil**
**4 drops helichrysum essential oil**

1. In a small bowl, combine all the ingredients. Whisk to blend thoroughly, and then transfer the blend to a small jar.

2. With a cotton swab, apply 1 drop of the blend to the boil. Repeat as often as needed, especially after bathing or showering.

STORAGE If you like, you can keep this gel in the refrigerator for an intense cooling sensation upon application; otherwise, keep in a cool, dark place.

# BRONCHITIS

With a painful cough, sore throat, and shortness of breath caused by swollen bronchial tubes, bronchitis can make you feel miserable. Antibiotics might be necessary, so see your doctor. Aromatherapy treatments can help by easing breathing and providing gentle comfort.

## Allspice-Sweet Orange Diffusion

Makes 1 treatment

Allspice and sweet orange help ease breathing while killing bacteria. Because allspice is a very spicy oil that can irritate mucous membranes, don't inhale directly from the diffuser.

**1 drop allspice essential oil**
**3 drops sweet orange essential oil**

1. Add the essential oils to your diffuser according to the manufacturer's instructions.

2. Run the diffuser nearby for 30 minutes three to four times daily until recovered.

SUBSTITUTION TIP If you don't have sweet orange essential oil on hand, you can use bergamot instead.

## Anise-Caraway Seed Vapor

Makes 1 treatment

Anise and caraway seed essential oils are potent antibacterial agents; they also provide a calming influence while helping expel phlegm.

1 cup steaming hot water
1 drop anise essential oil
2 drops caraway seed essential oil

1. Pour the water into a large mug, and then add the essential oils.

2. Hold the mug in front of you and occasionally breathe in the vapors as you relax. Continue until the water cools. Repeat two to three times daily until recovered.

## Soothing Spearmint-Hyssop Gargle

Makes 8 ounces

Hyssop and spearmint essential oils offer antiseptic and expectorant properties, which help bring comfort and promote healing.

7 ounces distilled water
1 ounce unflavored vodka
3 drops hyssop essential oil
2 drops spearmint essential oil

1. In a bottle or jar, combine all the ingredients. Shake well to blend, and then shake again before each use.

2. Gargle with 1 tablespoon of the blend for 30 seconds, being careful not to swallow. Spit out when finished. Repeat two to three times daily until recovered.

# BRUISES

Often painful and always colorful, bruises occur when trauma causes blood vessels located just beneath the skin's surface to break. Aromatherapy treatments don't make bruises disappear overnight, but they do promote faster healing.

## Hyssop-Lavender Balm

Makes 50 treatments

Hyssop and lavender improve circulation and promote faster healing while providing pain relief. This handy roll-on makes a convenient addition to your first aid kit.

1 tablespoon calendula oil
   or sweet almond oil
16 drops lavender essential oil
12 drops hyssop essential oil

1. In a small bottle, preferably with a roll-on applicator, combine all the ingredients. Shake well to blend.

2. With your fingertips or the roller, apply 3 to 4 drops of the blend to the bruise, using a little more or less as needed to cover the affected area. Repeat two to three times daily until the bruise is gone.

STORAGE Keep in a convenient location if you plan to use it up within a few weeks; otherwise, keep in a cool, dark place for up to a year.

## Helichrysum Compress

Makes 1 treatment

Helichrysum essential oil brings quick pain relief and promotes healing, while a cold compress helps take the sting out of a fresh bruise and minimize swelling. If your bruise is more than two or three hours old, apply a warm compress or heating pad instead.

**1 drop carrier oil**
**1 drop helichrysum essential oil**

1. With your fingertips or a cotton swab, apply the carrier oil to the bruise, and then apply the helichrysum essential oil. Use another drop or two of each oil if the bruise is very large.

2. Wrap an ice pack in a hand towel and lay it over the bruise. Leave the compress in place for 30 minutes, removing it periodically if your skin starts to feel uncomfortably numb.

## Chamomile-Rose Balm

Makes 1 ounce

Softly scented chamomile and rose blend with jojoba and coconut oil to ease inflammation and promote faster healing.

**1½ tablespoons coconut oil, softened**
**½ tablespoon jojoba oil**
**4 drops Roman or German chamomile**
**1 drop rose otto or rose absolute**

1. In a small bowl, combine all the ingredients. Whisk to blend thoroughly, and then transfer the balm to a small jar.

2. Apply a pea-size amount to the bruise, using a little more or less as needed to cover the bruise completely, and gently massage the area. Repeat two to three times daily until the bruise is gone.

SUBSTITUTION TIP If you don't have rose oil, use 4 drops of lavender instead.

# BUNIONS

When the bones in the big toe are out of alignment, pain, inflammation, and even arthritis can result. Aromatherapy can help bring relief, especially when combined with ice, heat, and/or massage.

## Tagetes Bunion Balm

Makes 1 ounce

Tagetes essential oil brings relief by targeting inflammation. This is a very powerful oil, and if you have sensitive skin, you should double the amount of carrier oil in the recipe.

**1 ounce jojoba oil**
**8 drops tagetes essential oil**

1. In a small bottle or jar, combine the oils. Shake well to blend.

2. Apply 1 drop of the blend to each bunion, and gently massage the area, using circular strokes. Also massage the arch of your foot, focusing on the forward portion.

## Frankincense Cold Compress

Makes 1 treatment

Frankincense essential oil relieves discomfort by targeting inflammation, while a cold compress helps minimize swelling.

**1 drop carrier oil**
**1 drop frankincense essential oil**

1. Elevate your foot. With your fingertips or a cotton ball, apply the carrier oil to the bunion, and then apply the frankincense essential oil.

2. Wrap the ice pack in a hand towel and lay it over the bunion. Leave the compress in place for 10 to 20 minutes, removing it periodically if your skin starts to feel uncomfortably numb.

## Copaiba-Peppermint Foot Cream

Makes about 4 ounces

Copaiba and peppermint essential oils combine with rich emollients to offer deep, penetrating pain relief and improve circulation while moisturizing feet.

**2 ounces coconut oil, melted**
**1 ounce shea butter**
**1 tablespoon sweet almond oil**
**1 tablespoon beeswax, melted**
**12 drops copaiba essential oil**
**8 drops peppermint essential oil**

1. In a large bowl, combine all the ingredients. Whisk to blend thoroughly.

2. Pour the blend into a jar and allow it to cool completely before capping.

3. Wash your feet, and then pat them dry. Apply a dime-size amount of the blend to each foot, and massage lightly.

# BURNS

Aromatherapy treatments are appropriate for first-degree burns. If you have a large second-degree burn with blisters, or if a third-degree burn has damaged skin and underlying tissue, seek emergency medical treatment.

## Lavender Neat Treatment

Makes 1 treatment

When applied immediately after a minor burn takes place, lavender essential oil helps stop pain and speed healing. Be sure to conduct a patch test before using this neat treatment.

**1 drop lavender essential oil**

1. Gently wash the burn with cold water, and then pat it dry.

2. Drip the essential oil onto the burn. Repeat every 2 to 3 hours until pain stops.

## Lavender-Geranium Compress

Makes 1 treatment

Lavender and geranium essential oil come together with healing aloe and a cold compress to relieve pain and improve healing.

½ teaspoon aloe vera gel
2 drops lavender essential oil
1 drop geranium essential oil

1. In a small bowl, combine all the ingredients. Stir well to blend.

2. Apply the entire blend to the burn. Wrap the ice pack in a soft cloth and lay it over the burn. Leave the pack in place for 5 to 10 minutes, or longer if needed. Repeat the treatment every 2 to 3 hours, up to three times daily.

## Chamomile-Tea Tree Balm

Makes about 1 ounce

Chamomile and tea tree essential oils can help older burns heal faster while preventing infection. This balm works best when applied after one of the first aid treatments described previously.

1 ounce fractionated coconut oil
12 drops Roman or German chamomile essential oil
6 drops tea tree essential oil

1. In a small bottle or jar, combine all the ingredients. Shake well to blend.

2. With a cotton swab, apply 1 drop of the blend to the burn. Repeat two to three times daily until recovered.

# CANKER SORES

Also known as aphthous ulcers, canker sores develop along the base of the gums and throughout the soft tissues of the mouth, appearing as small, red bumps that burst, leaving shallow yellowish or white lesions behind.

## Tea Tree Rinse

Makes about 4 ounces

Tea tree essential oil brings quick pain relief and helps prevent canker sores from becoming infected.

3½ ounces distilled water
1 tablespoon fractionated coconut oil
8 drops tea tree essential oil

1. In a bottle or jar, combine all the ingredients. Shake well to blend, and then shake again before each use.

2. Rinse your mouth with 1 teaspoon of the blend for 30 seconds to 1 minute, focusing on the area where canker sores are present, being very careful not to swallow the mixture. Spit out when finished. (Flush the drain with hot water.) Repeat two to three times daily until recovered.

## Dill Seed Balm

Makes 1 ounce

Dill seed essential oil helps canker sores by easing pain and speeding healing. Although some sources state that this oil is edible, it is best to avoid swallowing it.

**1 ounce fractionated coconut oil**
**10 drops dill seed essential oil**

1. In a small bottle or jar, combine the ingredients. Shake well to blend.

2. With a cotton swab, apply 1 drop of the blend to the canker sore. Use a new swab for each sore. Repeat the treatment once or twice daily until recovered.

## Oregano Salve and Compress

Makes 1 tablespoon

Oregano essential oil relieves discomfort and helps prevent infection by killing bacteria. Because this oil can irritate mucous membranes, it must be heavily diluted before using on canker sores.

**1 tablespoon fractionated coconut oil**
**1 drop oregano essential oil**

1. In a small bottle or jar, combine the ingredients. Shake well to blend.

2. Apply 1 drop of the blend to a cotton ball or a piece of gauze, and then position it over the canker sore.

3. Hold the compress in place for 3 to 4 minutes. Repeat the treatment two to three times daily until recovered.

# CARPAL TUNNEL SYNDROME

The discomfort carpal tunnel sufferers feel is caused by pressure on the nerve that provides movement and feeling to various parts of the hand. Serious cases often warrant surgery, but you can use a combination of aromatherapy and improved ergonomics to relieve minor cases.

## Minty Thyme-Rosemary Balm

Makes about 8 ounces

Peppermint, thyme, and rosemary essential oils offer deep penetration to bring quick, lasting relief. As a bonus, this balm moisturizes hands and smells divine.

2 ounces coconut oil, melted
2 ounces beeswax, melted
2 ounces shea butter
2 ounces sweet almond oil
40 drops peppermint essential oil
20 drops thyme essential oil
10 drops rosemary essential oil

1.  In a large bowl, combine all the ingredients. Use an electric hand mixer or whisk to blend thoroughly.

2.  Pour the blend into a jar and allow it to cool completely before capping.

3.  Apply a dime-size amount of the blend to the affected hand and wrist, and massage the area, using light strokes. Repeat two to three times daily as needed.

## Clove Bud, Black Pepper, and Ginger Soak

Makes 1 treatment

Clove bud, black pepper, and ginger essential oils combine with Epsom salt to penetrate deeply, targeting inflammation and providing quick relief.

1 gallon hot water
1 tablespoon Epsom salt
1 teaspoon fractionated coconut oil
3 drops black pepper essential oil
3 drops ginger essential oil
1 drop clove bud essential oil

1. In a large bowl or basin large enough to accommodate your hand and wrist, combine all the ingredients.

2. Position yourself comfortably and soak the painful area for 10 to 15 minutes. Repeat daily as needed.

## Juniper Berry, Lavender, and Thyme Compress

Makes about 1 tablespoon

Juniper berry, lavender, and thyme bring relief by increasing circulation and targeting inflammation. A warm or hot compress intensifies the effect.

1 tablespoon fractionated coconut oil
12 drops juniper berry essential oil
12 drops lavender essential oil
12 drops thyme essential oil

1. In a small bottle or jar, combine all the ingredients. Shake well to blend.

2. Apply ½ teaspoon of the blend to the affected hand and wrist, using a little more or less as needed, and massage the area.

3. Cover the area with a warm heating pad according to the manufacturer's instructions. Leave the heating pad in place for 10 to 15 minutes. Repeat daily as needed.

# CHICKEN POX

Chicken pox is caused by the varicella-zoster virus, and manifests as itchy, painful blisters that can eventually cover the entire body. Aromatherapy doesn't cure chicken pox, but treatments do provide some much-needed relief from discomfort.

## Lavender-Tea Tree Milk Bath

Makes 4 treatments

Added to comforting powdered goat milk, lavender and tea tree essential oils soothe irritation and help compromised skin heal.

2 cups powdered goat milk
20 drops lavender essential oil
10 drops tea tree essential oil

1. In a large bowl, combine all the ingredients. Whisk to blend thoroughly.

2. Sift the powder into a second bowl to break up any lumps, and then transfer the blend to a jar.

3. Draw a warm bath and add ½ cup of the blend to the tub, using your hand to stir it in. Soak in the bath for 15 to 20 minutes. Repeat once daily until recovered.

## Oregano-Thyme Powder

**Makes about 8 ounces**

Oregano and thyme essential oils help prevent infection and soothe itching. If you're not fond of the smell, you can replace these oils with lavender and tea tree.

10 drops oregano essential oil
10 drops thyme essential oil
4 ounces baking soda
4 ounces non-GMO cornstarch
1 teaspoon of uncooked rice
    (optional, for humidity control)

1. In a large measuring cup, combine the essential oils and the baking soda. Stir well to combine.

2. Sift the mixture into a large bowl, and then add the cornstarch. Whisk to blend thoroughly. If you live in a humid climate, add the rice to keep the powder from clumping, and mix in well. Transfer the blend to a glass or metal sugar shaker.

3. Sprinkle 1 teaspoon of powder onto the palm of your hand, and then apply to the affected body parts. Use a little more or less as needed, and repeat two to three times daily until recovered.

## Synergistic Chicken Pox Blend

**Makes about 2 ounces**

Tea tree, sandalwood, lavender, clove bud, and geranium soothe itching and help prevent infection while chicken pox heals.

2 ounces fractionated coconut oil
10 drops lavender essential oil
10 drops sandalwood essential oil
10 drops tea tree essential oil
5 drops clove bud essential oil
5 drops geranium essential oil

1. In a small bottle or jar, combine all the ingredients. Shake well to blend.

2. With a cotton ball, apply ½ teaspoon of the blend to each affected area, using a little more or less as needed to cover all the pox. Repeat two to three times daily until recovered.

# COLDS

Chest congestion, coughing, and stuffy or runny noses are all symptoms of the common cold— for which there is no known cure. Aromatherapy brings relief without the unpleasant side effects that often accompany drugstore remedies.

## Bay Laurel-Lavender Diffusion

Makes 1 treatment

Bay laurel is a powerful antiseptic and anti-spasmodic essential oil that can help purify the air in your home while providing relief from coughing and congestion. Too much can irritate mucous membranes, however, so don't breathe directly from the diffuser.

**2 drops bay laurel essential oil**
**1 drop lavender essential oil**

1. Add the essential oils to your diffuser according to the manufacturer's instructions.

2. Run the diffuser nearby. Repeat two to three times daily.

## Caraway-Clove Bud
## Chest Rub

Makes about 8 ounces

Caraway and clove bud bring relief from relentless coughing and congestion via their antispasmodic and expectorant properties. As a bonus, this blend smells a bit nicer than classic eucalyptus-based rubs.

2 ounces coconut oil, melted
2 ounces shea butter
1 ounce sweet almond oil
1 ounce beeswax, melted
25 drops clove bud essential oil
25 drops caraway essential oil

1. In a large bowl, combine all the ingredients. Whisk to blend thoroughly.

2. Pour the blend into a jar and allow it to cool completely before capping.

3. With your fingertips, apply a dime-size amount of the blend to the chest, and massage the area, using light strokes. Repeat two to three times daily as needed.

## May Chang-Lemon Lotion

Makes about 8 ounces

May Chang and lemon offer some protection from viruses and bacteria, and this blend promotes a clear airway.

8 ounces unscented body lotion
  or hand cream
20 drops lemon essential oil
10 drops May Chang essential oil

1. In a large bowl, combine all the ingredients. Whisk to blend thoroughly, and then transfer the lotion to a jar or back to its original container.

2. Apply 1 teaspoon of the blend to your hands, arms, and shoulders. Use a little more or less as needed, and feel free to apply the lotion to other body parts. Use as often as you like throughout the day, especially after washing your hands.

STORAGE Keep this lotion in a convenient location if you plan to use it all within two weeks; otherwise, keep it in a glass bottle or jar in a cool, dark place.

# COLD SORES

Also known as fever blisters, cold sores are caused by the herpes simplex virus, and are extremely contagious. Aromatherapy treatments don't cure the virus, but they do provide relief and can sometimes shorten the duration of an outbreak.

## Soothing Niaouli-Hops Balm

Makes about 1 ounce

Niaouli and hops, together with fractionated coconut oil, help bring quick comfort to cold sores while promoting faster healing.

1 ounce fractionated coconut oil
10 drops hops essential oil
10 drops niaouli essential oil

1. In a small bottle or jar, combine all the ingredients. Shake well to combine.

2. With a cotton swab, apply 1 drop of the blend to each affected area, using a new cotton swab for each area. Repeat two to three times daily.

## Synergistic Cold Sore Ointment

Makes 1 ounce

Tea tree, peppermint, lavender, and lemon essential oils work together to bolster your immune system and keep a cold sore from growing larger.

1 ounce coconut oil, softened
3 drops lavender essential oil
2 drops tea tree essential oil
2 drops lemon essential oil
1 drop peppermint essential oil

1. In a small bowl, combine all the ingredients. Whisk to blend thoroughly, and then transfer the ointment to a small jar.

2. With a cotton swab, apply 1 drop of the blend to the cold sore, using a new swab for each affected area. Repeat three to four times daily.

## Melissa Neat Treatment

Makes 1 treatment

Melissa is a potent antiviral essential oil that can help shorten the duration of a cold sore. Applying it at the first sign of a telltale tingle can keep an outbreak to a minimum. Be sure to conduct a patch test before using this neat treatment.

1 drop melissa essential oil

3. With a cotton swab, apply the melissa essential oil to the affected area.

4. Use a new swab for each affected area. Repeat three to four times daily.

SUBSTITUTION TIP If you don't have melissa essential oil, try 1 drop of lavender instead.

# COLIC

Some signs of colic include inconsolable crying that can last for more than three hours, a hard, gassy tummy, and lots of kicking. Aromatherapy can bring temporary relief, but you'll still need to determine and address the causes of your baby's discomfort.

## Synergistic Colic Blend

Makes about 4 ounces

Digestive essential oils such as cardamom, ginger, and fennel seed bring relief from gas and cramping so that your baby can relax.

4 ounces jojoba oil
12 drops cardamom essential oil
12 drops fennel seed essential oil
12 drops ginger essential oil
12 drops lavender essential oil
8 drops spearmint essential oil
8 drops German or Roman chamomile essential oil

1. In a bottle or jar, combine all the ingredients. Shake well to blend.

2. Warm your hands by rubbing them together vigorously. Apply 2 drops of the blend to the baby's lower back, and massage the blend in, using light, gentle strokes.

3. Turn your baby over and apply 1 drop of the blend to the bottom of each foot, again massaging gently.

4. Just before dressing the baby, apply 2 drops of the blend to the baby's abdomen using light, clockwise strokes. Repeat two to three times daily as needed.

## Soothing Lavender Diffusion

Makes 1 treatment

Lavender essential oil is safe for your baby, and it promotes peaceful sleep while also helping other family members to relax.

**3 drops lavender essential oil**

1. Add the essential oils to your diffuser according to the manufacturer's instructions.
2. Run the diffuser in the area where the baby spends lots of time. Repeat as needed.

## Catnip-Fennel Seed Bath Blend

Makes about 2 ounces

Catnip and fennel seed are classic ingredients in oral colic treatments, but don't try to treat this ailment by administering these oils by mouth. A warm, soothing bath provides safe, gentle relief.

**2 ounces jojoba oil**
**10 drops lavender essential oil**
**5 drops catnip essential oil**
**3 drops fennel seed essential oil**

1. In a small bottle or jar, combine all the ingredients. Shake well to blend.
2. Fill baby's bathtub with warm water and add 2 drops of the blend. Bathe your baby as usual, and then pat him or her dry. Follow up with a soothing massage using the Synergistic Colic Blend (page 90), if you like. Repeat once daily.

SUBSTITUTION TIP If you don't have catnip and fennel seed, increase the amount of lavender to 20 drops.

# CONCENTRATION

Work, study, and even driving in traffic all call for a high level of focus. Aromatherapy helps by stimulating memory and promoting alertness.

## Rosemary-Lemon Hand Cream

Makes about 4 ounces

A blend of rosemary and lemon makes for an irresistible fragrance that doubles as an aromatherapy treatment to promote concentration.

4 ounces unscented hand cream
   or body butter
30 drops lemon essential oil
16 drops rosemary essential oil

1. In a large bowl, combine all the ingredients. Whisk to blend thoroughly, and then transfer the cream to a bottle or jar.

2. Apply 1/2 teaspoon to the palm of one hand, and then massage the blend into your skin while inhaling deeply. Repeat as often as you like.

SUBSTITUTION TIP If you plan to spend time in the sun, replace the lemon essential oil with 10 drops of peppermint.

## Basil, Rosemary, and Cypress Diffusion

Makes 1 treatment

This fragrant blend makes your home or office smell fantastic, and it improves your ability to work or study.

3 drops cypress essential oil
2 drops basil essential oil
1 drop rosemary essential oil

1. Add the essential oils to your diffuser according to the manufacturer's instructions.
2. Run the diffuser nearby. Repeat as needed.

## Grapefruit-Spearmint Spritz

Makes about 4 ounces

This fantastic blend calls for grapefruit and spearmint essential oils, which stimulate concentration while promoting a positive outlook. This blend also makes a fragrant room spray.

4 ounces distilled water
30 drops grapefruit essential oil
20 drops spearmint essential oil

1. In a bottle with a fine-mist spray top, combine all the ingredients. Shake well to blend, and then shake again before each use.
2. Apply 1 spritz of the blend to your hair or skin, or mist your clothing instead if you plan to be in the sun. Repeat as often as you like.

# CONGESTION

Often caused by allergies or experienced alongside common cold symptoms, congestion prevents you from breathing comfortably. Aromatherapy treatments help by thinning out mucus and promoting an open airway.

## Caraway Seed-May Chang Shower Steam

Makes 1 treatment

Potent caraway seed and May Chang essential oils combine with your shower's steam to deliver quick relief from congestion.

**6 drops May Chang essential oil**
**3 drops caraway seed essential oil**

1. Apply the essential oils to a folded washcloth and position it on the shower floor, opposite the area where you stand.

2. Enjoy a hot, steamy shower and breathe deeply while your sinuses open. Repeat the treatment once or twice daily while dealing with congestion.

SUBSTITUTION TIP If you don't have these essential oils on hand, use 9 drops of eucalyptus or peppermint instead.

## Copaiba-Spanish Sage Vapor

Makes 1 treatment

Copaiba and Spanish sage essential oils work together to open your airway. This is a pungent-smelling treatment, but it provides quick relief.

2 cups steaming hot water
1 drop copaiba essential oil
1 drop Spanish sage essential oil

1. Pour the water into a large bowl, and then add the essential oils. Place a box of tissues nearby.

2. Sit comfortably in front of the bowl and drape a towel over your head and the bowl, creating a tent that concentrates the steam and vapors. Emerge to blow your nose or breathe cool air as needed. Try to spend 10 minutes with the treatment, and repeat it once or twice daily while you are recovering.

## Soothing Spruce-Yuzu Massage

Makes 1 ounce

Spruce and yuzu essential oils target bacteria while offering a clean, bracing fragrance that improves your mood while helping you breathe better.

1 ounce sweet almond oil
3 drops spruce essential oil
6 drops yuzu essential oil

1. In a small bottle or jar, combine all the ingredients. Shake well to blend.

2. With your fingertips or a cotton ball, apply 1/2 teaspoon of the blend to your chest and throat. Repeat two to three times daily until recovered.

SUBSTITUTION TIP If you plan to spend time in the sun, replace the yuzu essential oil with 2 drops of peppermint or 4 drops of spearmint.

PREFERENCE TIP Add an additional drop of spruce for a more woody scent or an additional 2 drops of yuzu for a more citrusy scent.

# CONSTIPATION

Changes in routine, lack of dietary fiber, and not enough exercise are just a few causes of constipation. Aromatherapy helps by improving circulation and gently encouraging smooth muscle tissue in the digestive tract to function properly.

## Synergistic Bath Blend

Makes 8 treatments

Lemon, basil, and black pepper essential oils promote circulation, while hot water and Epsom salt encourage your muscles to relax.

4 cups Epsom salt
1 tablespoon sweet almond oil
16 drops lemon essential oil
8 drops basil essential oil
8 drops black pepper essential oil

1.  In a large bowl, combine all the ingredients. Stir well to combine.

2.  Draw a hot bath and add ½ cup of the blend. Spend at least 15 minutes soaking. Repeat daily while suffering from constipation.

## Rosemary-Sweet Orange Compress

Makes 1 treatment

Rosemary and sweet orange essential oils promote relaxation and increase circulation, while heat promotes further relaxation.

½ teaspoon carrier oil
8 drops sweet orange essential oil
4 drops rosemary essential oil

1. In a small bowl, combine all the ingredients. Stir well to combine.

2. With your fingertips or a cotton ball, apply the entire treatment to your lower abdomen, focusing on the area located 2 inches below your navel.

3. Lie on your back and cover your abdomen with a warm heating pad, following the manufacturer's instructions for safe use. Relax for at least 15 minutes. Repeat once or twice daily while suffering from constipation.

## Peppermint-Fennel Seed Lotion

Makes 1 treatment

Peppermint and fennel seed stimulate the digestive tract and increase circulation, bringing relief from discomfort.

1 teaspoon unscented body lotion
4 drops peppermint essential oil
6 drops fennel seed essential oil

1. In the palm of your hand, combine all the ingredients.

2. Apply the blend to your lower abdomen, and massage the area, using clockwise strokes. Rest for at least 15 minutes, if possible. Repeat once or twice daily while suffering from constipation.

# CUTS AND SCRAPES

Kitchens, backyards, and playgrounds are hot spots for cuts and scrapes. Simple aromatherapy treatments help prevent infection while easing pain and promoting healing.

## Lavender Neat Treatment

Makes 1 treatment

Lavender essential oil soothes minor cuts and scrapes quickly while serving as a natural antiseptic and helping skin heal faster. Be sure to conduct a patch test before using this undiluted treatment.

**1 drop lavender essential oil**

1. Wash the wound and pat it dry.
2. Apply the lavender essential oil by dripping it directly onto the wound from the bottle, being careful not to touch the bottle to the wound. Use another drop or two if you have a large cut and need additional coverage.

## Tagetes-Rosewood Balm

Makes about 2 ounces

Tagetes and rosewood essential oils provide analgesic and antiseptic properties that combine to bring relief from pain while helping prevent infection.

1 ounce coconut oil, melted
1 tablespoon beeswax, melted
1 tablespoon sweet almond oil
10 drops rosewood essential oil
10 drops tagetes essential oil

1. In a medium bowl, combine all the ingredients. Whisk to blend thoroughly.

2. Pour the blend into a jar and allow it to cool completely before capping.

3. Wash the affected area and gently pat it dry. With your fingertips or a cotton swab, apply a pea-size amount of the blend to the wound and allow it to melt in. Repeat two to three times daily as needed.

## Patchouli-Myrrh Antiseptic Gel

Makes about 4 ounces

Patchouli and myrrh smell marvelous, but that's not all: These essential oils help minor wounds heal faster while preventing infection.

4 ounces 100 percent pure aloe vera gel
8 drops myrrh essential oil
6 drops patchouli essential oil

1. In a medium bowl, combine all the ingredients. Whisk to blend thoroughly, and then transfer the gel to a jar.

2. Wash the affected area and gently pat it dry. With your fingertips or a cotton swab, apply a pea-size amount of the blend to the wound and allow it to melt in. Repeat two to three times daily as needed.

# DIAPER RASH

A painful, angry-looking diaper rash can happen despite your best efforts to keep your infant dry. Aromatherapy treatments help soothe the sting and promote healing, and they're completely nontoxic.

## Lavender-Roman Chamomile Cleansing Wipes

Makes 80 to 100 disposable wipes

Healing lavender and Roman chamomile essentials come together with aloe to soothe irritated skin while leaving your baby fresh and clean.

1 roll premium paper towels
2 cups distilled water
1 tablespoon natural baby shampoo
1 tablespoon aloe vera gel
1 tablespoon organic olive oil
10 drops lavender essential oil
10 drops Roman chamomile essential oil

1. With a sharp plain-edge knife, cut the paper towel roll in half horizontally.

2. In a large bowl, combine all the ingredients. Stir well.

3. Place one half of the paper towel roll into the bowl, allowing the roll to absorb some of the liquid. Flip the roll over to ensure even absorption. Repeat the process with the other half of the paper towel roll.

4. Pull the cardboard cores out of the center of each roll to allow you to pull wipes up from the center. Place each roll of wipes in a one-gallon plastic zip-top bag.

5. Use as needed, as you would other cleansing wipes, during diaper changes.

## Frankincense-Myrrh
## Barrier Cream

Makes 4 ounces

Soothing frankincense and myrrh blend with rich coconut oil to stop bacteria while providing a light layer of protection from moisture.

2 ounces coconut oil, melted
2 ounces shea butter
4 drops frankincense essential oil
4 drops myrrh essential oil

1. In a medium bowl, combine all the ingredients. Whisk to blend thoroughly, and then transfer the cream to a jar. Allow it to cool completely before capping.

2. With your fingertips or a cotton ball, apply ½ teaspoon of the cream to the baby's diaper region. Use a little more or less, ensuring that you spread a thin layer over the entire affected area. Repeat treatment at each diaper change.

PREFERENCE TIP If you would prefer a much thicker barrier cream, replace the coconut oil and shea butter with 4 ounces of softened lanolin.

## Lavender-Neroli
## Baby Powder

Makes 4 ounces

Calming lavender and neroli combine with naturally absorbent arrowroot powder to prevent the accumulation of excess moisture and stop bacteria from spreading, without the dangers associated with the use of talcum powder.

4 ounces arrowroot powder
4 drops lavender essential oil
2 drops neroli essential oil
1 teaspoon of uncooked rice
   (optional, for humidity control)

1. In a large bowl, combine all the ingredients. Whisk to blend thoroughly.

2. Sift the mixture into a second bowl to remove any lumps. Transfer the blend to a glass or metal sugar shaker. Add the rice (if using).

3. After each diaper change, apply ½ teaspoon of powder to the baby's diaper area, covering the barrier cream. Use a little more or less to ensure that you've left a thin coat of powder on all vulnerable surfaces.

SUBSTITUTION TIP If you don't have neroli essential oil, use 2 drops of Roman chamomile or 6 drops of the lavender.

# DIARRHEA

With the cramping and frequent, watery stools, diarrhea can make you feel miserable. Aromatherapy can bring some relief by calming inflammation and cramping, but it's important to stay dehydrated and avoid trigger foods.

## Copaiba-Coriander Compress

Makes 1 treatment

Copaiba and coriander combine with soothing heat to reduce spasms and bring comfort to an overworked digestive system.

½ teaspoon fractionated coconut oil
1 drop copaiba essential oil
1 drop coriander essential oil

1. In the palm of your hand, combine all the ingredients.

2. Apply the blend to your lower abdomen, and gently massage the area in a clockwise direction.

3. Lie down and cover your lower abdomen with a warm heating pad, following the manufacturer's instructions for safe use. Leave the heating pad in place for at least 15 minutes. Repeat two to three times daily while suffering from diarrhea.

## Triple Spice Massage Blend

Makes 1 ounce

Ginger, cinnamon leaf, and clove bud essential oils soothe your digestive system and increase circulation, helping you recover faster from a bout of diarrhea.

1 ounce fractionated coconut oil
4 drops ginger essential oil
2 drops cinnamon leaf essential oil
2 drops clove bud essential oil

1. In a small bottle or jar, combine all the ingredients. Shake well to blend.

2. Apply ½ teaspoon of the blend to your lower abdomen, focusing on the area located about 2 inches below the navel, and massage the area, using light clockwise strokes.

3. Relax and breathe deeply, while sipping ginger or chamomile tea (if you have some available). Repeat two to three times daily while suffering from diarrhea.

## Synergistic Abdominal Massage Blend

Makes 2 ounces

Ravensara leaf, *Eucalyptus radiata*, lavender, and marjoram essential oils combine to attack bacteria while improving circulation and relieving discomfort.

2 ounces fractionated coconut oil
4 drops lavender essential oil
4 drops marjoram essential oil
2 drops *Eucalyptus radiata* essential oil
2 drops ravensara leaf essential oil

1. In a bottle or jar, combine all the ingredients. Shake well to blend.

2. Apply ½ teaspoon of the blend to your abdomen. With the navel as the center starting point, gently massage the area, using clockwise strokes. Use a little more or less oil as needed, ensuring that you cover the entire abdomen. Repeat once or twice daily while suffering from diarrhea.

3. If you have time, cover your abdomen with a warm heating pad, following the manufacturer's instructions for safe use. Leave the heating pad in place for 15 minutes.

# EARACHE/ SWIMMER'S EAR

Earaches and swimmer's ear involve the middle and outer ear, rather than the very sensitive inner ear. Aromatherapy treatments bring relief, but be sure to see your doctor if you suspect an infection.

## Eucalyptus Radiata-Rosemary Massage

Makes 1 treatment

Eucalyptus and rosemary essential oils fight bacteria and help prevent infection. Do not place the oils directly in the ear canal.

6 drops carrier oil
2 drops *Eucalyptus radiata* essential oil
2 drops rosemary essential oil

1. Apply 2 drops of carrier oil to the area extending from the back of the corner of your jaw, and extend the line to the front of the throat, all the way down to your collarbone. Repeat on the other side of your neck, even if only one ear is involved.

2. Apply 1 drop of *Eucalyptus radiata* essential oil to each side of your head and neck, covering the carrier oil. Wait for 1 minute.

3. Apply 1 drop of rosemary essential oil to each side of your head and neck, following the same path as before and covering the *Eucalyptus radiata* essential oil.

4. Immediately after applying the rosemary essential oil, apply 1 more drop of carrier oil on each side, following the same path as before.

5. Repeat the treatment morning and night for 3 days, and then continue only at night until all discomfort is gone.

## Oregano Earache Treatment

Makes 1 treatment

The smell of oregano essential oil is reminiscent of pizza, but don't let that fool you. It's a potent agent in the battle against bacteria.

1 drop carrier oil
1 drop oregano essential oil

1. Apply the carrier oil and oregano essential oil to a cotton ball.

2. Lie on your side with the affected ear facing the ceiling. Nestle the cotton ball into the outer portion of your ear and leave it in place for 15 minutes. Repeat twice daily while earache persists.

## Lavender Neat Treatment

Makes 1 treatment

Lavender essential oil kills bacteria while helping ease the discomfort that accompanies swimmer's ear. Apply the essential oil only to the outer portion of your ear. Be sure to conduct a patch test before using this undiluted treatment.

1 drop lavender essential oil

1. Wash the affected ear and pat it dry.

2. With your fingertip, apply 1 drop of lavender essential oil to the outer portion of your ear. Repeat two to three times daily while discomfort persists.

# ECZEMA

Itchy, inflamed skin calls for gentle treatment. Aromatherapy treatments can help resolve redness and discomfort inside the elbows, on the backs of the knees, and other places where eczema tends to appear.

## Soothing Palmarosa-Lavender Bath Salts

Makes 8 treatments

Lavender and palmarosa essential oils ease inflammation, especially when combined with warm water and Epsom salt.

1 tablespoon fractionated coconut oil
16 drops lavender essential oil
8 drops palmarosa essential oil
4 cups Epsom salt

1. In a large bowl, combine the fractionated coconut oil and the essential oils. Add the Epsom salt and stir well to blend. Transfer the bath salts to a jar.

2. Draw a warm (not hot) bath and dissolve ½ cup of the bath salts in the water. Soak in the bath for at least 15 minutes. Repeat two to three times weekly while working to resolve eczema.

## Geranium-Lavender Balm

Makes about 4 ounces

Geranium and lavender soothe irritation and promote healing. Coconut oil is particularly soothing, because it has anti-inflammatory properties of its own.

4 ounces coconut oil, softened
32 drops lavender essential oil
16 drops geranium essential oil

1. In a medium bowl, combine all the ingredients. Whisk to blend thoroughly, and then transfer the balm to a jar.

2. With your fingertips, apply a pea-size amount to each affected area, using a little more or less as needed to leave a thin layer of the balm on the skin.

CHILD-FRIENDLY TIP If you are making this balm for a child less than six years old, omit the geranium essential oil.

## Cooling Oregano-Cucumber Seed Spray

Makes about 4 ounces

Brisk oregano and cucumber seed essential oils combine with soothing aloe and refreshing witch hazel to ease the itching and inflammation that accompanies eczema.

2 ounces distilled water
1 ounce alcohol-free witch hazel
1 ounce aloe vera gel
12 drops cucumber seed essential oil
3 drops oregano essential oil

1. In a bottle with a fine-mist spray top, combine all the ingredients. Shake well to blend, and then shake again before each use.

2. Apply 1 spritz to each patch of eczema. Repeat twice daily.

# EXHAUSTION

Exhaustion can take a serious toll on your mental and physical health, compounding other issues and making everything seem more difficult. Aromatherapy can help lessen the impact while you address the root cause.

## Uplifting Citrus-Basil Diffusion

Makes 1 treatment

Crisp, cheerful citrus essential oils improve your mood, while basil acts as a strong mental stimulant. This blend smells delightful, making it enjoyable in your home or at the office.

1 drop basil essential oil
1 drop grapefruit essential oil
1 drop lemon essential oil
1 drop mandarin essential oil

1. Add the essential oils to your diffuser according to the manufacturer's instructions.

2. Run the diffuser nearby. Repeat two to three times daily as needed.

## Rosemary-Peppermint Temple Rub

Makes 150 treatments

Soothing rosemary and invigorating peppermint come together with a touch of tangy lemon to create a wonderfully uplifting scent that sharpens your mind while improving your mood.

1 tablespoon sweet almond oil
20 drops lemon essential oil
10 drops peppermint essential oil
4 drops rosemary essential oil

1. In a small bottle, preferably with a roll-on applicator, combine all the ingredients. Shake well to blend.

2. With your fingertips or the roller, apply 1 drop of the blend to each of your temples, and gently massage the area. Repeat two to three times daily.

SUBSTITUTION TIP If you plan to spend time in the sun, omit the lemon essential oil from this blend, or wear a hat that blocks the sun from hitting your temples.

STORAGE Keep in a convenient location if you plan to use it up within a few weeks; otherwise, keep in a cool, dark place for up to a year.

## Basil-Geranium Shower Steam

Makes 1 treatment

Uplifting basil and geranium essential oils combine with your shower's steam to deliver quick relief from exhaustion while elevating your mood.

6 drops geranium essential oil
2 drops basil essential oil

1. Apply the essential oils to a folded washcloth and position it on the shower floor, opposite the area where you stand.

2. Enjoy a hot, steamy shower and breathe deeply while you lather up with your favorite soap. Repeat the treatment once daily while coping with exhaustion.

SUBSTITUTION TIP If you don't have these essential oils on hand, use 2 drops of rosemary and 3 drops of peppermint instead.

# FEVER

While a fever is an expression of your body's natural defense against infection, it can make you feel quite uncomfortable. Aromatherapy treatments bring relief, but use good judgment by consulting your doctor to determine when medical intervention might be necessary.

## Cool Spearmint Compress

Makes 1 treatment

Bracing spearmint essential oil combines with cold water to bring comfort and help cool your fever.

½ cup distilled water
2 ice cubes
2 drops spearmint essential oil

1. In a small bowl, pour the distilled water over the ice cubes, and then add the spearmint essential oil.

2. Soak a folded washcloth in the solution, and then place it on your forehead. Top the washcloth with a folded hand towel to catch any drips.

3. Leave the compress in place for 15 minutes. Repeat as needed.

## Aromatic Eucalyptus Sponge Bath

Makes 1 treatment

Cool eucalyptus essential oil brings rapid relief from a fever's heat. Adults can use lemon eucalyptus or *Eucalyptus globulus*; seniors and children tolerate *Eucalyptus radiata* better.

2 cups of ice water
2 drops eucalyptus essential oil

1. In a bowl, combine the ice water and eucalyptus essential oil. Soak a washcloth or body sponge in the mixture and wring it out so that it doesn't drip.

2. Run the washcloth or sponge across the forehead, the back of the neck, the armpits, and the chest. Wet the sponge again when it becomes warm and reapply. Repeat every 3 to 4 hours.

## Cooling Peppermint Body Wrap

Makes 1 treatment

Refreshing peppermint essential oil combines with water and a clean sheet to create a cooling body wrap that helps bring body temperature down.

2 cups ice water
2 drops peppermint essential oil

1. In a large bowl or basin, combine the ice water and the peppermint essential oil.

2. Place a folded sheet into the bowl or basin and allow it to absorb the water. Flip the sheet over to ensure that both sides are coated.

3. Wring out any excess water, and then unfold the sheet. Wrap it around the entire body, ensuring that the sheet makes contact with the skin.

4. Relax while sitting or lying on a few towels. Leave the wrap in place for at least 15 minutes, and repeat two to three times over the course of a day.

# FIBROMYALGIA

Fibromyalgia brings a number of distressing symptoms with it, including muscle pain, fatigue, and headaches. Aromatherapy helps by soothing discomfort while addressing stress and improving your emotional state.

## Eucalyptus, Juniper, and Geranium Lotion

Makes about 8 ounces

Penetrating eucalyptus, woody juniper, and fragrant geranium combine to ease discomfort and bolster your immune system while promoting a positive mood.

8 ounces unscented body lotion
16 drops geranium essential oil
8 drops eucalyptus essential oil
8 drops juniper essential oil

1. In a large bowl, combine all the ingredients. Whisk to blend thoroughly, and then transfer the lotion to a jar or back to its original container.

2. Apply 1 teaspoon of the blend to your hands, arms, shoulders, and other body parts as desired, using a little more or less as needed. Repeat as often as you like throughout each day, especially after washing your hands.

STORAGE Keep this lotion in a convenient location if you plan to use it all within two weeks; otherwise, keep it in a glass bottle or jar in a cool, dark place.

## Spicy Frankincense-Helichrysum Balm

Makes about 4 ounces

Clove bud, frankincense, and helichrysum essential oils offer analgesic properties that target pain and help relax tight muscle fibers.

2 ounces shea butter
1 ounce coconut oil, melted
1 tablespoon beeswax, melted
1 tablespoon sweet almond oil
20 drops clove bud essential oil
12 drops frankincense essential oil
12 drops helichrysum essential oil

1. In a large bowl, combine all the ingredients. Whisk to blend thoroughly.

2. Pour the blend into a jar and allow it to cool completely before capping.

3. Apply a pea-size amount of the balm to each painful point, and massage the area, using light strokes. Repeat once or twice daily, using a little more or less as needed to bring relief.

## Minty Lemon-Lavender Temple Rub

Makes 150 treatments

Brisk peppermint and bright lemon come together with a touch of lavender to ease pain and stress while offering an uplifting scent.

12 drops peppermint essential oil
20 drops lemon essential oil
20 drops lavender essential oil

1. In a small bottle, preferably with a roll-on applicator, combine all the ingredients. Shake well to blend.

2. With your fingertips or the roller, apply 1 drop of the blend to each of your temples. This treatment can also be applied to sore spots. Repeat as needed.

STORAGE Keep in a convenient location if you plan to use it up within a few weeks; otherwise, keep in a cool, dark place for up to a year.

# FLATULENCE

Believe it or not, the average person passes gas somewhere between 13 and 21 times daily. When gas is stinky or painful, or you're suffering from nonstop flatulence, aromatherapy can help.

## Soothing Peppermint-Melissa Massage

*Makes about 2 ounces*

Peppermint and melissa increase circulation and enhance digestion, helping stop discomfort and reducing flatulence.

1 tablespoon coconut oil, melted
1 tablespoon hemp oil
1 tablespoon shea butter
1 tablespoon sweet almond oil
16 drops melissa oil
12 drops peppermint essential oil

1. In a medium bowl, combine all the ingredients. Whisk to blend thoroughly, and then transfer the balm to a small jar.

2. Apply 1 teaspoon of balm to the abdomen, and massage the area, using firm clockwise strokes. Repeat as needed.

## Coriander-Dill Seed Compress

Makes 1 treatment

Copaiba and dill seed combine with soothing heat to soothe painful intestinal spasms and bring comfort to your digestive system.

½ teaspoon fractionated coconut oil
1 drop coriander essential oil
1 drop dill seed essential oil

1. In the palm of your hand, combine all the ingredients.
2. Apply the blend to your lower abdomen, and gently massage the area in a clockwise direction.
3. Lie down and cover your lower abdomen with a warm heating pad, following the manufacturer's instructions for safe use. Leave the heating pad in place for at least 15 minutes. Repeat two to three times daily while suffering from severe flatulence.

## Warming Ginger-Anise Bath Salts

Makes 8 treatments

Warm cinnamon leaf, ginger, chamomile, and anise essential oils combine with Epsom salt to ease gas pains by relaxing smooth muscle tissue and encouraging flatulence to subside.

2 tablespoons fractionated coconut oil
2 drops cinnamon leaf essential oil
4 drops anise essential oil
10 drops ginger essential oil
10 drops Roman chamomile essential oil
4 cups Epsom salt

1. In a large bowl, combine the fractionated coconut oil and the essential oils. Add the Epsom salt and stir well to blend. Transfer the bath salts to a jar.
2. Draw a hot bath and add ½ cup of bath salts. Soak in the bath for at least 15 minutes. Repeat once daily while dealing with painful flatulence.

# FLU

"Flu" is a generic term for various strains of influenza virus. Severe cases call for immediate medical intervention, but when common symptoms such as low fever, body aches, and congestion are present, aromatherapy brings relief.

## Palmarosa-Palo Santo Massage

Makes about 4 ounces

Fragrant palmarosa and palo santo essential oils offer antiviral and antibacterial properties, plus they cool fevers and provide relief to stiff, sore muscles.

2 ounces shea butter
1 ounce coconut oil, melted
1 tablespoon beeswax, melted
1 tablespoon sweet almond oil
20 drops palmarosa essential oil
20 drops palo santo essential oil

1. In a large bowl, combine all the ingredients. Whisk to blend thoroughly.

2. Pour the blend into a jar and allow it to cool completely before capping.

3. With your fingertips, apply a dime-size amount of the blend to your chest and throat. You can also apply a drop of the blend to areas where muscle soreness is worst. Repeat two to three times until recovered.

## Citrus Bay-Spanish Sage Bath Salts

Makes 8 treatments

Delectable yuzu, spicy bay laurel, and Spanish sage essential oils combine with Epsom salt to fight infection and promote clear breathing.

2 tablespoons fractionated coconut oil
12 drops Spanish sage essential oil
12 drops bay laurel essential oil
24 drops yuzu essential oil
4 cups Epsom salt

1. In a large bowl, combine the fractionated coconut oil with the essential oils. Add the Epsom salt and stir well to blend. Transfer the bath salts to a jar.

2. Draw a hot bath and add ½ cup of bath salts. Soak in the bath for at least 15 minutes while breathing deeply. Repeat once daily while fighting the flu.

SUBSTITUTION TIP If you plan to spend time in the sun, replace the yuzu with 12 drops of spearmint essential oil.

## Peppermint-Eucalyptus Shower Melts

Makes 10 treatments

Peppermint and eucalyptus essential oils bring quick relief from congestion, especially when used in a hot, steamy shower. It's easy to double or triple this recipe so you have plenty of treatments on hand when you need them most.

2½ cups baking soda
½ cup water
20 drops peppermint essential oil
30 drops eucalyptus essential oil

1. Preheat the oven to 350°F, and line a muffin tin with 10 cupcake liners.

2. In a small bowl, combine baking soda and water. Stir into a thick paste.

3. Evenly divide the paste between the cupcake liners, and bake for 20 minutes or until dry.

4. Allow the melts to cool completely, and then peel the liners off. To each melt, add 2 drops of peppermint and 3 drops of eucalyptus oil. Transfer the melts immediately to a wide-mouth jar or storage container and seal.

5. Place 1 melt in the shower stall just before stepping in. Breathe deeply while you enjoy the fragrant steam. Repeat once or twice daily while recuperating from the flu.

# FOLLICULITIS

Folliculitis is a particularly nasty rash that is characterized by inflamed hair follicles. Whether chemical irritation, infection, or skin trauma is to blame, aromatherapy treatments can bring relief and help the skin heal.

## Lavandin Balm

Makes about 4 ounces

Lavandin essential oil is a comforting antiseptic that also offers pain relief. Coconut oil offers antibacterial properties, too.

**4 ounces fractionated coconut oil**
**20 drops lavandin essential oil**

1. In a bottle or jar, combine the ingredients. Shake well to blend.

2. Apply 1 teaspoon of the blend to the affected area, using a little more or less as needed. Repeat twice daily until folliculitis clears.

## Lemon Verbena-Lavender Gel

Makes about 4 ounces

Lemon verbena and lavender combine to stop infection and ease inflammation. Aloe vera gel provides comfort and promotes healing.

3½ ounces aloe vera gel
1 tablespoon fractionated coconut oil
20 drops lavender essential oil
12 drops lemon verbena essential oil

1. In a large bowl, combine all the ingredients. Whisk to blend thoroughly, and then transfer the gel to a jar.

2. Apply 1 teaspoon of the blend to the affected area, using a little more or less as needed. Repeat two to three times daily until folliculitis clears.

STORAGE If you like, you can keep this gel in the refrigerator for an intense cooling sensation upon application; otherwise, keep in a cool, dark place.

## Soothing Myrtle Spray

Makes about 8 ounces

Myrtle essential oil helps open pores, and it acts as a potent disinfectant, which makes it a great remedy for this skin condition.

4 ounces witch hazel
3½ ounces distilled water
1 tablespoon fractionated coconut oil
20 drops myrtle essential oil

1. In a bottle with a fine-mist spray top, combine all the ingredients. Shake well to blend, and then shake again before each use.

2. Apply 1 spritz to the affected area. Use a little more if needed, and repeat twice daily until folliculitis clears.

# GASTRIC REFLUX

Gastric reflux, the symptoms of which include heartburn, nausea, and regurgitation, happens when intra-abdominal pressure causes acidic stomach contents to back up into the esophagus. Aromatherapy offers temporary relief, but it's important to address the root cause, as gastroesophageal reflux disease may be the culprit.

## Peppermint-Lime Chest Rub

Makes about 1 ounce

Peppermint and lime work together to relax smooth muscle tissues and provide temporary relief from gastric reflux symptoms.

1 ounce fractionated coconut oil
6 drops peppermint essential oil
12 drops lime essential oil

1. In a small bottle or jar, combine all the ingredients. Shake well to blend.
2. Apply ½ teaspoon of the mixture to your chest, beginning at the bottom of the sternum and working your way up toward your throat. Repeat once daily or as needed.

## Fennel Seed-Ginger Compress

Makes 1 treatment

Licorice-scented fennel seed and warm ginger combine with soothing heat to relax the abdomen and relieve some of the burning.

½ teaspoon fractionated coconut oil
2 drops ginger essential oil
1 drop fennel seed essential oil

1. In the palm of your hand, combine all the ingredients.
2. Apply the blend to your upper abdomen, and gently massage the area in a clockwise direction.
3. Lie on your left side, and cover your upper abdomen with a warm heating pad, following the manufacturer's instructions for safe use. Leave the heating pad in place for at least 15 minutes. Repeat two to three times daily while working to resolve gastric reflux.

## Lemon Drop

Makes 1 treatment

When followed by a swish of saliva, a drop of lemon on your tongue signals your stomach to temporarily halt acid production. Most of the lemon is absorbed by your mouth, and the saliva neutralizes the remainder.

1 drop lemon essential oil

1. With a pipette or dropper, drip the lemon essential oil onto your tongue.
2. Swish your entire mouth with saliva, and then swallow the saliva. Repeat up to twice daily as needed.

# HALITOSIS

Spicy food, sinus infections, and dry mouth are a few of the many things that can lead to halitosis. Aroma-therapy treatments work wonders for bad breath and cost far less than their commercial counterparts.

## Lavender-Spearmint Breath Spray

*Makes 4 ounces*

Lavender and spearmint kill bacteria while leaving you with fresh, fragrant breath. You can replace the vodka in this recipe with additional distilled water if you'd prefer an alcohol-free breath spray.

**3½ ounces distilled water**
**1 tablespoon unflavored vodka**
**1 drop lavender essential oil**
**3 drops spearmint essential oil**
**3 drops liquid stevia**

1. In a bottle with a fine-mist spray top, combine all the ingredients. Shake well to blend, and then shake again before each use.

2. Apply 1 spritz to the inside of your mouth. Repeat as often as needed to keep breath smelling fresh.

## Citrus-Clove Bud Breath Drops

Makes 150 treatments

Sweet orange, grapefruit, and clove bud essential oils combine to target bacteria and leave you with fresh-smelling breath.

1 tablespoon fractionated coconut oil
2 drops grapefruit essential oil
2 drops sweet orange essential oil
1 drop clove bud essential oil

1. In a small bottle with an orifice reducer, combine all the ingredients. Shake well to blend.

2. Apply 1 drop of the blend to the underside of your tongue directly from the bottle, being careful not to touch the bottle to your mouth. Repeat as needed to keep bad breath at bay.

SUBSTITUTION TIP If you prefer a minty scent, replace the citrus and clove bud essential oils with 5 drops of spearmint.

STORAGE Keep in a convenient location if you plan to use it up within a few weeks; otherwise, keep in a cool, dark place for up to a year.

## Lavender Mouthwash

Makes 4 ounces

Lavender essential oil makes short work of bacteria, leaving your breath with a pleasant fragrance. If the flavor of lavender doesn't appeal to you, this mouthwash can also be made with lemon or spearmint.

3½ ounces distilled water
1 tablespoon brandy
4 drops lavender essential oil

1. In a bottle or jar, combine all the ingredients. Shake well to blend, and then shake again before each use.

2. Swish your mouth with ½ tablespoon of the blend for 30 seconds to 1 minute, being careful not to swallow. Spit out when finished. Repeat two to three times daily.

# HANGOVER

When you've indulged in a few too many drinks, your pounding head and churning stomach can make it difficult to face the day ahead. Aromatherapy can help by promoting detoxification, restoring your sense of balance, and helping your head feel clearer.

### Citrus-Mint Diffusion

Makes 1 treatment

Cheerful citrus and fresh peppermint helps you clear the cobwebs from your head, plus they provide some relief from nausea.

1 drop lemon essential oil
1 drop peppermint essential oil
1 drop sweet orange essential oil

Add the essential oils to your diffuser according to the manufacturer's instructions. Run the diffuser nearby. Repeat as needed throughout the day.

SUBSTITUTION TIP If you like, you can try other citrus scents such as bergamot, lime, grapefruit, or mandarin in this blend.

## Detoxifying Massage Oil

Makes about 4 ounces

Soothing lavender, crisp citrus, and cooling peppermint combine to cheer you up and support the detoxification process. Be sure to drink lots of water throughout the day.

4 ounces fractionated coconut oil
20 drops lavender essential oil
20 drops lemon essential oil
20 drops mandarin essential oil
20 drops peppermint essential oil

1. In a bottle or jar, combine all the ingredients. Shake well to blend.

2. Apply 1 teaspoon of the blend to your chest, arms, and shoulders, and lightly massage the areas of application while breathing deeply. Then massage 1 drop of the oil into each of your temples.

## Restorative Shower Melts

Makes 10 treatments

Bracing basil, soothing patchouli, and comforting lavender, lemon, and peppermint essential oils bring you back to your senses, especially when combined with a hot, steamy shower.

2½ cups baking soda
½ cup water
10 drops basil essential oil
20 drops lavender essential oil
20 drops peppermint essential oil
20 drops patchouli essential oil
30 drops lemon essential oil

1. Preheat the oven to 350°F, and line a muffin tin with 10 cupcake liners.

2. In a small bowl, combine baking soda and water. Stir into a thick paste.

3. Evenly divide the paste between the cupcake liners, and bake for 20 minutes or until dry.

4. Allow the melts to cool completely, and then peel the liners off. To each melt, add 1 drop of basil, 2 drops of lavender, 2 drops of peppermint, 2 drops of patchouli, and 3 drops of lemon. Transfer the melts immediately to a wide-mouth jar or storage container and seal.

5. Place 1 melt in the shower stall just before stepping in. Breathe deeply while you enjoy the fragrant steam. Repeat once or twice daily while recovering from a hangover.

# HAY FEVER/ ALLERGIES

Sneezing, watery eyes, and a familiar itchy feeling in your airway tell you that hay fever or allergies are at work. Some aromatherapy treatments help block the histamines that cause your symptoms, while others address discomfort directly.

## Niaouli Inhaler

Makes 1 treatment

Niaouli essential oil is an excellent decongestant that clears your head while improving your mood and giving your immune system a boost.

**20 drops niaouli essential oil**

1. Apply the essential oil to the cotton wick of the aromatherapy inhaler.

2. Hold the inhaler beneath your nose, and inhale slowly through both nostrils to a count of five. Hold your breath for another count of five, and then exhale slowly. Repeat as needed to prevent and soothe symptoms.

**SUBSTITUTION TIP** If you don't have an inhaler, you can transfer the blend to a small, dark glass bottle and inhale directly from the bottle, or place 3 drops of the niaouli in your diffuser.

## Breathe-Easy Synergistic Blend

Makes 150 treatments

Refreshing eucalyptus, peppermint, and copaiba come together with crisp cypress to clear your head and relieve respiratory symptoms.

1 tablespoon fractionated coconut oil
12 drops copaiba essential oil
12 drops cypress essential oil
10 drops *Eucalyptus globulus* essential oil
8 drops peppermint essential oil

1. In a small bottle, preferably with a roll-on applicator, combine all the ingredients. Shake well to blend.

2. With your fingertips or the roller, apply 1 drop to the pulse point behind each of your ears, and gently massage the areas, drawing the blend toward the front of your throat.

3. Apply 1 drop of the blend to the base of your throat, and gently massage the area. Repeat every 2 hours as needed.

STORAGE Keep in a convenient location if you plan to use it up within a few weeks; otherwise, keep in a cool, dark place for up to a year.

## Melissa-Chamomile Diffusion

Makes 1 treatment

Melissa and Roman chamomile essential oils offer antihistamine properties that lessen the impact allergens have on your body.

2 drops Roman chamomile essential oil
1 drop melissa essential oil

Add the essential oils to your diffuser according to the manufacturer's instructions. Run the diffuser nearby. Repeat as needed throughout the day.

SUBSTITUTION TIP If you are allergic to daisies, Roman chamomile may make your symptoms worse rather than better; omit the chamomile and diffuse 3 drops of melissa instead.

# HEAD LICE

Head lice are tiny, parasitic insects that spend their lives feeding on blood drawn from the scalp. Lice are highly contagious; even the cleanest individual can get them from contact with an infested person or from contact with items that have come into contact with an infested individual's head.

## Cinnamon Leaf-Tea Tree Shampoo

Makes about 4 ounces

Cinnamon leaf and tea tree essential oils combine to create a strong insecticide that kills head lice and eggs. Be absolutely certain to conduct a patch test before using this potent recipe. Cinnamon bark essential oil hasn't been proven effective, so be sure to use the correct oil in this recipe.

2 ounces unscented shampoo
2 ounces rubbing alcohol
24 drops cinnamon leaf essential oil
24 drops tea tree essential oil

1. In a plastic squeeze bottle, combine all the ingredients. Stir well with a thin utensil.

2. Wet hair and apply ½ tablespoon of shampoo to the hair and scalp, using a little more or less to ensure that the entire head is covered. Scrub well and leave the shampoo in place for 10 to 15 minutes.

3. Rinse the shampoo out while running a delousing comb through your hair to remove dead lice, then check for remaining lice.

4. It is advisable to follow up with Geranium Conditioning Treatment (page 129). Repeat the treatment again in 1 week. Watch carefully for signs of reinfestation.

## Oregano Delousing Rinse

Makes 1 treatment

When diluted in rubbing alcohol, oregano essential oil has been shown to kill 100 percent of adult lice and eggs. This spicy oil can cause irritation in sensitive individuals, so be sure to conduct a patch test before using this remedy.

2 ounces rubbing alcohol
12 drops oregano essential oil

1. In a plastic squeeze bottle, combine the ingredients. Shake well to blend.

2. Wet hair and apply the entire treatment to the hair and scalp, ensuring that the entire head is covered. Leave the treatment in place for 10 to 15 minutes.

3. Rinse the treatment out while running a delousing comb through your hair to remove dead lice, then check for remaining lice.

4. It is advisable to follow up with Geranium Conditioning Treatment. Repeat the treatment again in 1 week. Watch carefully for signs of reinfestation.

## Geranium Conditioning Treatment

Makes 1 treatment

Geranium is less potent than other insecticidal essential oils, but it does kill lice, especially when left on hair overnight. As a bonus, it nourishes and heals skin while conditioning hair.

1 tablespoon jojoba oil
10 drops geranium essential oil

1. In the palm of your hand, combine the ingredients. Rub your hands together to distribute the treatment evenly.

2. Apply the conditioner to the hair and scalp, and then use a fine comb to ensure that the entire head has been treated. Cover the head with a soft cap, such as a knit winter hat, before going to bed.

3. In the morning, shampoo your hair as usual and then comb out any remaining lice and/or nits. Repeat the treatment again in 1 week. Watch carefully for signs of reinfestation.

# HEADACHE

Stress, tension, and dehydration are among the top causes of headaches. Aromatherapy treatments help ease the pain while you determine the root cause of the headache and address it.

## Lavender, Marjoram, and Basil Balm for Tension Headaches

Makes 100 treatments

Warming basil, marjoram, and lavender help tight head and neck muscles relax, easing the pain and allowing you to relax.

1 tablespoon fractionated coconut oil
18 drops lavender essential oil
12 drops marjoram essential oil
6 drops basil essential oil

1. In a small bottle, preferably with a roll-on applicator, combine all the ingredients. Shake well to blend.

2. With your fingertips or the roller, apply 1 drop to each of your temples, and gently massage the areas while breathing deeply.

3. Apply 2 to 3 drops of the blend to the base of your neck, and massage the area. If you can pinpoint any sore spots on your head, apply 1 drop to each of them, as well.

STORAGE Keep in a convenient location if you plan to use it up within a few weeks; otherwise, keep in a cool, dark place for up to a year.

## Rosemary, Basil, and Mint Shower Melts for General Headaches

Makes 10 treatments

Bracing rosemary, basil, and peppermint essential oils relieve headaches quickly, especially when combined with the steam from your hot shower.

2½ cups baking soda
½ cup water
10 drops rosemary essential oil
10 drops basil essential oil
20 drops peppermint essential oil

1. Preheat the oven to 350°F, and line a muffin tin with 10 cupcake liners.

2. In a small bowl, combine baking soda and water. Stir into a thick paste.

3. Evenly divide the paste between the cupcake liners, and bake for 20 minutes or until dry.

4. Allow the melts to cool completely, and then peel the liners off. To each melt, add 1 drop of rosemary, 1 drop of basil, and 2 drops of peppermint essential oil. Transfer the melts immediately to a wide-mouth jar or storage container and seal

5. Place 1 melt in the shower stall just before stepping in. Breathe deeply while you enjoy the fragrant steam. Repeat once or twice daily while dealing with headaches.

## Rosemary-Eucalyptus Vapor for Sinus Headaches

Makes 1 treatment

Rosemary and eucalyptus essential oils work together to open your airway, take the pressure off your sinuses, and stop your pain. This is a relaxing treatment, but you'll feel wide awake afterward.

2 cups steaming hot water
1 drop rosemary essential oil
1 drop eucalyptus essential oil (any species)

1. Pour the water into a large bowl, and then add the essential oils. Place a box of tissues nearby.

2. Sit comfortably in front of the bowl and drape a towel over your head and the bowl, creating a tent that concentrates the steam and vapors. Emerge to blow your nose or breathe cool air as needed. Try to spend 10 minutes with the treatment, and repeat it once or twice daily while dealing with sinus headaches.

# HEARTBURN

Heartburn occurs when stomach acid travels back up into the esophagus, usually after you've eaten a rich or spicy meal. Aromatherapy can cool the burn and make you more comfortable, but it's best to avoid trigger foods and overeating altogether—long-term exposure to stomach acid will damage your esophagus.

## Spearmint Compress

Makes 1 treatment

Cool spearmint essential oil combines with soothing heat to ease discomfort and stop any feelings of nausea that accompany heartburn.

**½ teaspoon fractionated coconut oil**
**4 drops spearmint essential oil**

1. In the palm of your hand, combine the ingredients.
2. Apply the blend to your upper abdomen, and gently massage the area in a clockwise direction.
3. Lie down and cover your upper abdomen with a warm heating pad, following the manufacturer's instructions for safe use. Leave the heating pad in place for at least 15 minutes. Repeat two to three times daily while suffering from heartburn.

## Synergistic Heartburn Blend

Makes about 4 ounces

Anise, caraway, coriander, ginger, fennel seed, and peppermint essential oils combine to ease indigestion and stop the burn fast.

4 ounces fractionated coconut oil
20 drops ginger essential oil
20 drops peppermint essential oil
14 drops caraway essential oil
14 drops coriander essential oil
10 drops anise essential oil
8 drops fennel seed essential oil

1. In a bottle or jar, combine all the ingredients. Shake well to blend.

2. With your fingertips, apply 1 teaspoon of the blend to your upper abdomen, chest, and throat, and gently massage the areas.

3. Lie on your left side and relax for 15 minutes. Repeat once or twice daily while coping with heartburn.

SUBSTITUTION TIP Peppermint can make heartburn worse in some individuals. If that's the case for you, make this recipe with spearmint essential oil in place of the peppermint.

## Minty Fennel Seed-Eucalyptus Lotion

Makes about 4 ounces

Fennel seed, ginger, and eucalyptus increase circulation and enhance digestion, while spearmint helps ease discomfort. Try using this blend before meals as a preventive measure.

4 ounces unscented body lotion
16 drops fennel seed essential oil
16 drops ginger essential oil
12 drops spearmint essential oil
12 drops eucalyptus essential oil

1. In a medium bowl, combine all the ingredients. Whisk to blend thoroughly, and then transfer the lotion to a small jar.

2. Apply 1 teaspoon of lotion to the upper abdominal area, and massage upward toward the chest. Repeat two to three times daily or as needed.

STORAGE Keep this lotion in a convenient location if you plan to use it all within two weeks; otherwise, keep it in a glass bottle or jar in a cool, dark place.

# HEAT RASH

Also known as prickly heat, heat rash is a bumpy pink or red rash that typically develops on body parts that have been covered by clothing during hot, humid weather. If the rash is accompanied by chills and/or fever, or if you see swelling, pus, or other signs of infection, skip the aromatherapy treatments and get to the doctor.

## Frankincense-Galbanum Spray

Makes about 8 ounces

Soothing frankincense and galbanum essential oils ease itching and discomfort while helping compromised skin heal. Witch hazel helps cool the skin so you feel more comfortable.

4 ounces distilled water
4 ounces witch hazel
12 drops frankincense essential oil
12 drops galbanum essential oil

1. In a bottle with a fine-mist spray top, combine all the ingredients. Shake well to blend, and then shake again before each use.

2. Apply 1 spritz to each affected area every 2 to 3 hours until the heat rash resolves.

## Bergamot-Helichrysum Compress

Makes 1 treatment

Combined with cold water, bergamot and helichrysum can provide much-need relief by calming the itching and helping your skin heal faster.

½ cup distilled water
2 ice cubes
1 drop bergamot essential oil
1 drop helichrysum essential oil

1. In a small bowl, pour the distilled water over the ice cubes, and then add the essential oils.

2. Depending on the size of the affected area, soak a washcloth or hand towel in the solution, and place it over the rash. Top the washcloth or towel with a folded hand towel to catch any drips.

3. Leave the compress in place for 15 minutes. Allow your skin to air-dry after removal. Repeat as needed until the heat rash resolves.

## Bedtime Elemi-Hops Flower Bath Salts

Makes 8 treatments

Elemi and hops flower essential oils combine with Epsom salt to soothe inflammation and stop the itching, while promoting relaxation so you can get to sleep.

2 tablespoons fractionated coconut oil
16 drops elemi essential oil
12 drops hops flower essential oil
4 cups Epsom salt

1. In a large bowl, combine the fractionated coconut oil with the essential oils. Add the Epsom salt and stir well to blend. Transfer the bath salts to a jar.

2. Draw a lukewarm bath and add ½ cup of bath salts. Soak in the bath for at least 15 minutes. Repeat each evening until the rash is gone.

CHILD-FRIENDLY TIP If you are making this blend for a child less than six years old, replace the elemi with Roman chamomile, and replace the hops flower with lavender.

# HEMORRHOIDS

Pain, swelling, itching, and irritation are symptoms of swollen blood vessels in and around the rectum. Hemorrhoids can develop when you strain too much during bowel movements, as well as when you are pregnant or diagnosed with liver disease. Aromatherapy treatments bring relief and can help stop the swelling, but in severe cases, medical intervention may be the only answer.

## Lemon-Cypress Compress

Makes 1 treatment

Lemon and cypress help soothe inflammation and shrink swelling. When combined with cold water, they bring rapid relief from discomfort.

½ cup distilled water
2 ice cubes
4 drops lemon essential oil
4 drops cypress essential oil

1. In a small bowl, pour the water over the ice cubes, and then add the essential oils.

2. Roll a washcloth into a cylinder and soak it in the solution.

3. Lie flat on your stomach with a towel underneath your pelvic area to catch any drips. Position the rolled-up washcloth between the gluteus maximus muscles so that it is in contact with the inflamed tissue.

4. Leave the compress in place for 15 minutes. Allow your skin to air-dry after removal, and repeat as needed until hemorrhoids resolve.

## Roman Chamomile Salve for Bleeding Hemorrhoids

Makes 1 ounce

Antiseptic tea tree and Roman chamomile essential oils help prevent infection, ease pain, and soothe irritated skin, while the avocado oil calms inflammation.

1 ounce avocado oil
8 drops Roman chamomile essential oil
2 drops tea tree essential oil

1. In a small bottle or jar, combine all the ingredients. Shake well to blend.

2. Thoroughly cleanse the affected area. With a cotton cosmetic pad, apply ¼ teaspoon of the blend. Repeat after bathing, showering, and bowel movements.

## Neroli-Myrrh Wipes

Makes 80 to 100 disposable wipes

Neroli and myrrh essential oils come together with aloe and witch hazel to ease itching and soothe irritated skin while leaving you feeling fresh.

1 roll premium paper towels
1 cup distilled water
1 cup alcohol-free witch hazel
2 tablespoons aloe vera gel
1 tablespoon avocado oil
1 tablespoon fragrance-free liquid soap
10 drops neroli essential oil
20 drops myrrh essential oil

1. With a sharp plain-edge knife, cut the paper towel roll in half horizontally.

2. In a large bowl, combine all the ingredients. Stir well.

3. Place one half of the paper towel roll into the bowl, allowing the roll to absorb some of the liquid. Flip the roll over to ensure even absorption. Repeat the process with the other half of the paper towel roll.

4. Pull the cardboard cores out of the center of each roll to allow you to pull wipes up from the center. Place each roll of wipes in a one-gallon plastic zip-top bag.

5. Use wipes as needed, especially after bowel movements.

# HIGH BLOOD PRESSURE

When your blood pressure is elevated, your heart must work harder to pump blood throughout the body. Aromatherapy can help lower blood pressure, but you'll need to address other factors such as smoking, stress, lack of exercise, and obesity to see lasting change.

## Relaxing Lavender-Marjoram Bath

Makes 8 treatments

Lavender and marjoram essential oils combine with magnesium-rich Epsom salt to promote deep relaxation and help bring blood pressure down temporarily. Talk to your doctor to ensure that this treatment is suitable for your condition.

2 tablespoons fractionated coconut oil
16 drops lavender essential oil
32 drops marjoram essential oil
4 cups Epsom salt

1. In a large bowl, combine the fractionated coconut oil with the essential oils. Add the Epsom salt and stir well to blend. Transfer the bath salts to a jar.

2. Draw a warm bath and add ½ cup of bath salts. Soak in the bath for at least 15 minutes. Repeat once daily as often as you like.

## Lavender, Frankincense, and Geranium Layer Treatment

Makes 1 treatment

Lavender, frankincense, and geranium essential oils help bring blood pressure down and temporarily stabilize it. Layering the oils lets you enjoy different benefits than you receive from blending, so to get the intended benefit from this treatment, don't mix these oils together before application.

3 drops lavender essential oil
3 drops frankincense essential oil
3 drops geranium essential oil
3 drops carrier oil

1. Apply the lavender essential oil to the left portion of your chest, over your heart. Wait for 1 minute, and then layer the frankincense essential oil over the lavender essential oil. Wait for another minute, and then layer the geranium essential oil over the frankincense essential oil. Immediately following the geranium layer, cover the area with the carrier oil.

2. If possible, spend 30 minutes or so relaxing, either lying down or with your feet elevated. Repeat the treatment two times daily while working to change your lifestyle and bring your blood pressure down for good.

## Lavender-Tea Tree Salve

Makes about 4 ounces

Lavender and tea tree essential oils promote relaxation and bring on a sense of calm, helping bring high blood pressure down.

4 ounces sweet almond oil
32 drops lavender essential oil
32 drops tea tree essential oil

1. In a bottle or jar, combine all the ingredients. Shake to blend.

2. With your fingertips, apply ½ teaspoon of the blend to your heart area, and massage the salve in well while breathing deeply. Take 10 or 15 minutes to relax with your feet up. Repeat three times daily.

# HIVES

Sometimes caused by allergies or intense periods of stress, hives can be as small as the tip of a pen to several inches across, and they sometimes connect to form even larger areas of red, angry itchiness. Aromatherapy treatments bring toxin-free comfort quickly; if a fever is present, call your doctor.

## Soothing Myrrh Bath

Makes 8 treatments

Myrrh essential oil combines with baking soda to ease pain and inflammation, and help stop the intense, burning itch that often accompanies hives.

2 tablespoons fractionated coconut oil
32 drops myrrh essential oil
4 cups baking soda

1. In a large bowl, combine the coconut oil with the essential oil. Stir with a thin utensil to blend.

2. Add the baking soda, and whisk to blend thoroughly. Transfer the mixture to a jar.

3. Draw a lukewarm bath and add ½ cup of the bath blend. Soak in the bath for at least 15 minutes. Repeat once or twice daily until hives are gone.

## Roman Chamomile-Lavender Spritz

Makes about 8 ounces

Soothing lavender and Roman chamomile combine with astringent witch hazel to bring fast relief from itching.

4 ounces distilled water
4 ounces witch hazel
20 drops lavender essential oil
20 drops Roman chamomile essential oil

1. In a bottle with a fine-mist spray top, combine all the ingredients. Shake well to blend, and then shake again before each use.

2. Apply 1 spritz to each affected area every 1 to 2 hours as needed for itching.

## Calming Ravintsara Balm

Makes about 1 ounce

Ravintsara essential oil calms pain and itching, and helps compromised skin heal. Its aroma brings quick relaxation, so if stress is to blame for your hives, this is a very good treatment to try.

1 ounce fractionated coconut oil
36 drops ravintsara essential oil

1. In a small bottle or jar, combine the ingredients. Shake well to blend.

2. With a cotton ball, apply 1 drop of the blend to each affected area. Use a little more or less as needed to cover all hives.

CHILD-FRIENDLY TIP If you're making this blend for a child less than six years old, replace the ravintsara with lavender essential oil.

# IMPETIGO

Impetigo begins as a red area that's often painful and itchy, after which an amber-colored crust forms as the infected area weeps and oozes. Aromatherapy treatments help by killing the *Staphylococcus aureus* bacteria that cause this highly infectious illness.

## Tea Tree-Lavender Layer Treatment

Makes 1 treatment

Tea tree and lavender essential oils are suitable for neat application, plus they offer strong antibacterial action. Layering the oils lets you enjoy different benefits than you receive from blending, so to get the intended benefit from this treatment, don't mix these oils together before application.

**1 drop tea tree essential oil**
**1 drop lavender essential oil**

1. With a cotton swab, apply the tea tree essential oil to the affected area. Wait 1 minute, and then use another cotton swab to apply the lavender essential oil. Repeat the treatment on all affected areas once or twice daily.

2. Once the crust disappears, stop applying the tea tree and use 1 drop of lavender essential on the affected areas to help heal compromised skin.

## Lavender Compress

Makes 1 treatment

Lavender essential oil kills bacteria, and combined with cold water, it offers rapid pain relief. This gentle treatment is ideal for children who are too young to handle stronger essential oils.

1 cup distilled water
2 ice cubes
10 drops lavender essential oil

1. In a large bowl, pour the distilled water over the ice cubes, and then add the essential oil.

2. Using enough to cover each affected area, moisten individual pieces of paper towel in the solution.

3. Lay the paper towel pieces over the affected areas, and leave them in place for 15 minutes.

4. Discard the used paper towels immediately after use. Allow skin to air-dry after removal, and repeat three to four times daily until impetigo is gone.

## Synergistic Impetigo Blend

Makes about 1 ounce

A combination of ravensara leaf, thyme, tea tree, and myrrh essential oils kills bacteria and speeds healing. Plus, fractionated coconut oil has antibacterial properties of its own.

1 ounce fractionated coconut oil
15 drops ravensara leaf essential oil
15 drops tea tree essential oil
10 drops thyme essential oil
10 drops myrrh essential oil

1. In a small bottle or jar, combine all the ingredients. Shake well to blend.

2. After bathing, use a cotton swab to apply 1 drop of the blend to each affected area. Use a new cotton swab for each application. Repeat the treatment once or twice daily until impetigo is gone.

# IMPOTENCE

When the cause of impotence is stress, anxiety, or mild depression, aromatherapy can help by removing those negative feelings so that you can relax and enjoy intimacy. If the cause is physical, you will need to see your doctor for a stronger treatment.

## Jasmine Massage

Makes 1 treatment

Jasmine is a powerful sensual stimulant that evokes a positive, receptive mood. A pre-diluted jasmine oil is ideal for this treatment, as it is ready to use straight from the bottle. Ensure that your blend is made with *Jasminum officinale*.

**6 drops pre-diluted jasmine oil**

1. Apply the jasmine oil to the palm of your hand, and then rub your hands together while inhaling deeply.

2. Lightly massage your arms, shoulders, and neck. Repeat each evening as you relax and unwind.

## Rose Linen Spray

Makes 8 ounces

Rose addresses a wide range of emotional problems, including anger, depression, and stress. Plus, it imparts a sensual, romantic mood. If you choose a pre-diluted rose oil, ensure that it is made with *Rosa damascena*.

**8 ounces distilled water**
**4 drops rose otto or 24 drops**
  **pre-diluted rose oil**

1.  In a bottle with a fine-mist spray top, combine ingredients. Shake well to blend, and then shake again before each use.

2.  Apply 6 to 8 spritzes to areas such as pillows, comforters, sheets, and bedroom curtains. You can also spray your hair and body, if you like.

## Sandalwood Balm

Makes 150 treatments

Sandalwood offers an exotic, woody fragrance that reduces tension and creates a sense of calm happiness. This balm helps shake off the effects of a hectic day, allowing you to relax and enjoy intimate moments.

**1 tablespoon sweet almond oil**
**20 drops sandalwood essential oil**

1.  In a small bottle, preferably with a roll-on applicator, combine the ingredients. Shake well to blend.

2.  With your fingertips or the roller, apply 1 drop to the pulse point behind each of your ears, and gently massage the areas. If a stronger personal fragrance is desired, apply a drop to each wrist, your throat, or your inner elbows.

STORAGE  Keep in a convenient location if you plan to use it up within a few weeks; otherwise, keep in a cool, dark place for up to a year.

# INDIGESTION

Uncomfortable belching, nausea, and a general sense of digestive distress are some of the hallmarks of indigestion. Aromatherapy brings quick comfort; however, if your symptoms are persistent, check with your doctor to rule out an underlying illness.

## Comforting Clove Bud Compress

*Makes 1 treatment*

Clove bud essential oil relaxes the smooth muscles of the digestive tract and prevents nausea, gas, and uncomfortable spasms. A warm compress brings additional relief.

**1 teaspoon fractionated coconut oil**
**3 drops clove bud essential oil**

1. In the palm of your hand, combine the ingredients.

2. Apply the blend to your abdomen, and gently massage outward in a clockwise direction, beginning at the navel.

3. Lie down and cover your abdomen with a warm heating pad, following the manufacturer's instructions for safe use. Leave the heating pad in place for at least 15 minutes. Repeat once or twice daily while suffering from indigestion.

## Peppermint Massage

Makes 1 treatment

Peppermint relaxes the digestive muscles and increases circulation to help you get over indigestion quickly. If you're feeling a bit nauseous, this is a good treatment to try.

**2 drops peppermint essential oil**
**2 drops carrier oil**

1. Apply the peppermint essential oil directly to the area located just beneath the sternum.

2. Apply the carrier oil over the peppermint oil, and lightly massage the area. Repeat once or twice daily while suffering from indigestion.

## Cardamom Balm

Makes about 4 ounces

Cardamom enhances circulation and stimulates healthy digestion. If you have overindulged, give this simple treatment a try.

**4 ounces coconut oil, softened**
**32 drops cardamom essential oil**

1. In a medium bowl, combine the ingredients. Whisk to blend thoroughly, and then transfer the balm to a jar.

2. Apply 1 teaspoon of the mixture to the upper abdomen, and lightly massage the area, using clockwise motions. Repeat once or twice daily while suffering from indigestion.

# INGROWN TOENAIL

Trimming your toenails too short and following the curvature of the toe rather than cutting straight across sets the stage for ingrown toenails. Aromatherapy treatments and proper trimming can help in minor cases, but serious ingrown toenails sometimes require medical intervention.

## Lavender-Tea Tree Footbath

Makes 1 treatment

When combined with a softening footbath, lavender and tea tree essential oils help compromised skin heal while providing protection from infection.

1 gallon hot water
2 tablespoons Epsom salt
10 drops lavender essential oil
4 drops tea tree essential oil

1. In a shallow basin that's large enough to accommodate your foot, combine the hot water and the Epsom salt.

2. Add the essential oils to the basin, and then put the affected foot into the water.

3. Soak your foot for 10 minutes, and then pat it dry. Apply an additional drop of lavender essential oil to the ingrown toenail.

4. If possible, trim the toenail back at a very slight angle to relieve the pressure. If you're not able to trim the toenail, gently slide a piece of waxed dental floss between the nail and the skin and try to trim again. If this doesn't work, repeat the footbath treatment every 2 to 4 hours until you are able to trim the toenail and relieve the pressure.

## Healing Frankincense Balm

Makes 1 ounce

Frankincense helps stop inflammation while helping skin heal. This balm is a good one to use after successfully trimming back an ingrown toenail.

1 ounce fractionated coconut oil
10 drops frankincense essential oil

1. In a small bottle or jar, combine the ingredients. Shake well to blend.

2. With a cotton swab, apply 2 drops of the balm to the affected toenail. Allow the treatment to absorb before putting on socks or shoes. Repeat two to three times daily.

## Lemon Eucalyptus-Clove Bud Compress

Makes 1 treatment

A cold compress made with lemon eucalyptus and clove bud essential oils help stop infection, soothe pain, and soften skin so that you can trim an ingrown toenail more comfortably.

½ cup distilled water
2 ice cubes
4 drops clove bud essential oil
2 drops lemon eucalyptus essential oil

1. In a small bowl, pour the distilled water over the ice cubes, and then add the essential oils.

2. Soak a folded washcloth in the solution, and then place it on the affected toe. Rest your foot on a towel and top the washcloth with a folded hand towel to catch any drips.

3. Leave the compress in place for 15 minutes. Allow your skin to air-dry after removal, and repeat as needed until you are able to trim the ingrown toenail.

# INSECT BITES/ BEE STINGS

Some insects deliver tiny bites that can cause an irritating itch, while bees and wasps deliver a much more powerful punch. Aromatherapy treatments bring quick, reliable relief. If you are allergic to bees, seek medical attention immediately.

## Lavender-Peppermint Anti-Itch Spray

Makes about 4 ounces

Lavender and peppermint combine with apple cider vinegar to provide rapid relief from the itching caused by mosquito, gnat, and chigger bites.

4 ounces organic apple cider vinegar
24 drops lavender essential oil
16 drops peppermint essential oil

1. In a bottle with a fine-mist spray top, combine all the ingredients. Shake well to blend, and then shake again before each use.

2. Apply 1 spritz to each itchy area every 1 to 2 hours as needed.

STORAGE If you like, you can keep this spray in the refrigerator for an intense cooling sensation upon application; otherwise, keep in a cool, dark place.

## Lavender-Eucalyptus Bee Sting Relief

Makes 1 treatment

Lavender and eucalyptus essential oils provide pain relief and help prevent infection after a nasty bee sting. An ice pack on top reduces swelling.

2 drops carrier oil
1 drop lavender essential oil
1 drop eucalyptus essential oil (any species)

1. If the bee left behind a stinger, remove it with a pair of tweezers, and then wash and dry the affected area.

2. Apply 1 drop of carrier oil to the sting site, and then apply the lavender essential oil.

3. Wait for 1 minute, and then apply the eucalyptus essential oil. Immediately top it with another drop of carrier oil.

4. Cover the treatment with a soft cloth, and then apply an ice pack. Leave the ice pack in place for 15 minutes. Repeat the treatment every 2 to 3 hours until pain subsides.

## Chamomile-Lavender Gel

Makes 1 ounce

This soothing chamomile-lavender combo provides relief from itchy bug bites while helping diminish swelling and inflammation. Aloe helps quicken skin healing, too.

1 ounce 100 percent pure aloe vera gel
6 drops lavender essential oil
6 drops Roman or German chamomile essential oil

1. In a small bowl, combine all the ingredients. Whisk to blend thoroughly, and then transfer the gel to a jar.

2. With a cotton swab, apply 1 drop of the blend to each insect bite. Repeat two to three times daily until the swelling and itching have subsided.

# INSOMNIA

Instead of reaching for pharmaceuticals, give aromatherapy a try the next time sleeplessness takes over. These comforting remedies work best when you focus on relaxing. You can make natural sleep easier by turning off electronics an hour before bedtime.

## Valerian-Cedarwood Bedtime Balm

Makes about 4 ounces

Valerian essential oil promotes deep, peaceful sleep. Cedarwood tempers its intensely woody, earthy aroma, which some people dislike. Don't drink alcohol or use sleep aids alongside this treatment.

2 ounces coconut oil, melted
1 ounce shea butter
1 tablespoon beeswax, melted
1 tablespoon sweet almond oil
40 drops valerian essential oil
20 drops cedarwood essential oil

1. In a large bowl, combine all the ingredients. Whisk to blend thoroughly.

2. Pour the blend into a jar and allow it to cool completely before capping.

3. With your fingertips, apply a dime-size amount to your shoulder and neck area. Repeat once nightly as needed to assist with falling asleep.

PREFERENCE TIP Check the blend's aroma before allowing it to cool. If you dislike the fragrance, add 10 drops of lavender or lavandin essential oil.

## Spikenard-Rose Bath Salts

Makes 8 treatments

Spikenard and rose combine with soothing Epsom salt to promote deep relaxation. Spikenard is a highly effective sedative, so finish important tasks before enjoying this treatment.

2 tablespoons fractionated coconut oil
40 drops spikenard essential oil
4 drops rose otto or 20 drops
    pre-diluted rose oil
4 cups Epsom salt

1. In a large bowl, combine the fractionated coconut oil and the essential oils. Add the Epsom salt and stir well to blend. Transfer the bath salts to a jar.

2. Draw a hot bath and add ½ cup of bath salts. Soak in the bath for 15 to 20 minutes. Repeat nightly as needed.

## Lavender-Chamomile Nighttime Shower Melts

Makes 10 treatments

Lavender and Roman chamomile essential oils help you fall asleep quickly, especially when combined with the steam from your hot shower. This treatment is ideal for travel, or for anyone who doesn't care much for baths.

2½ cups baking soda
½ cup water
40 drops lavender essential oil
40 drops Roman chamomile essential oil

1. Preheat the oven to 350°F, and line a muffin tin with 10 cupcake liners.

2. In a small bowl, combine baking soda and water. Stir into a thick paste, evenly divide the paste between the cupcake liners, and bake for 20 minutes or until dry.

3. Allow the melts to cool completely, and then peel the liners off. To each melt, add 4 drops of lavender and 4 drops of Roman chamomile essential oil. Transfer the melts immediately to a wide-mouth jar or storage container.

4. Place 1 melt in the shower stall just before stepping in. Breathe deeply while you enjoy the fragrant steam. Repeat nightly as needed.

# IRRITABLE BOWEL SYNDROME (IBS)

Abdominal pain, nausea, bloating, and alternating bouts of constipation and diarrhea are among the most common symptoms of IBS, which is caused by uncoordinated muscle movements within the digestive tract. Be sure to obtain a diagnosis from your doctor before trying aromatherapy, because IBS shares symptoms with disorders that require medical intervention.

## Soothing Chamomile Balm

Makes about 2 ounces

Both Roman and German chamomile essential oil encourage smooth muscle tissue to relax, plus they enhance digestion, helping you obtain relief from your discomfort.

1 tablespoon coconut oil, melted
1 tablespoon sweet almond oil
1 tablespoon shea butter
1 tablespoon hemp oil
20 drops German or Roman chamomile essential oil

1. In a medium bowl, combine all the ingredients. Whisk to blend thoroughly, and then transfer the balm to a small jar.

2. Apply 1 teaspoon of balm to the abdomen, and massage the area, using firm clockwise strokes. Repeat two to three times daily as needed, whenever IBS symptoms cause discomfort.

## Mandarin-Neroli Diffusion

Makes 1 treatment

Stress often plays a role in IBS. Mandarin and neroli essential oils come together to create a relaxing yet cheerful scent that supports your mood while you deal with uncomfortable symptoms.

**2 drops mandarin essential oil**
**1 drop neroli essential oil**

Add the essential oils to your diffuser according to the manufacturer's instructions. Run the diffuser nearby. Repeat as often as you like.

## Peppermint-Fennel Seed Compress

Makes 1 treatment

Soothing peppermint and fennel seed essential oils combine with soothing heat to relax intestinal spasms and encourage better digestion.

**1 teaspoon fractionated coconut oil**
**2 drops peppermint essential oil**
**3 drops fennel seed essential oil**

1. In the palm of your hand, combine all the ingredients.
2. Apply the blend to your lower abdomen, and gently massage the area in a clockwise direction.
3. Lie down and cover your lower abdomen with a warm heating pad, following the manufacturer's instructions for safe use. Leave the heating pad in place for at least 15 minutes. Repeat two to three times daily when IBS symptoms flare up.

# JET LAG

Long flights that cross multiple time zones can leave you feeling disoriented and fatigued. Aromatherapy and some simple adjustments to your schedule a few days before travel can help minimize jet lag's effects.

## Bergamot-Citrus Shower Melts

Makes about 8 ounces

Bright, cheerful tangerine, grapefruit, and bergamot combine to clear mental cobwebs and heighten your senses to help you start the day off, or to revive and refresh you on a sleepy afternoon.

2½ cups baking soda
½ cup water
40 drops bergamot essential oil
20 drops tangerine essential oil
20 drops grapefruit essential oil

1. Preheat the oven to 350°F, and line a muffin tin with 10 cupcake liners.

2. In a small bowl, combine baking soda and water. Stir into a thick paste.

3. Evenly divide the paste between the cupcake liners, and bake for 20 minutes or until dry.

4. Allow the melts to cool completely, and then peel the liners off. To each melt, add 4 drops of bergamot, 2 drops of tangerine, and 2 drops of grapefruit essential oil. Transfer the melts immediately to a wide-mouth jar or storage container.

5. Place 1 melt in the shower stall just before stepping in. Breathe deeply while you enjoy the fragrant steam. Repeat daily as needed.

## Rosewood-Lemon Verbena Lotion

Makes about 8 ounces

Rosewood and lemon verbena help you de-stress while encouraging you to remain alert. If you plan to spend time in the sun, apply the lotion only to areas that will be covered by clothing.

8 ounces unscented body lotion
 or hand cream
20 drops lemon verbena essential oil
20 drops rosewood essential oil

1. In a large bowl, combine all the ingredients. Whisk to blend thoroughly, and then transfer the lotion to a jar or back to its original container.

2. Apply 1 teaspoon of the blend to your hands, arms, and shoulders. Use a little more or less as needed, and feel free to apply the lotion to other body parts. Use as often as you like throughout each day, especially after washing your hands.

STORAGE Keep this lotion in a convenient location if you plan to use it all within two weeks; otherwise, keep it in a glass bottle or jar in a cool, dark place.

## Minty Rosemary-Lemon Mist

Makes about 8 ounces

When jet lag has come for a visit, brisk peppermint, rosemary, and lemon essential oils combine to waken your senses and keep you feeling alert.

7 ounces distilled water
1 ounce witch hazel
15 drops lemon essential oil
10 drops peppermint essential oil
5 drops rosemary essential oil

1. In a bottle with a fine-mist spray top, combine all the ingredients. Shake well to blend, and then shake again before each use.

2. Apply 1 spritz to your pulse points or, if you will be in the sun, just spray your clothing or the air around you and inhale. Repeat as needed.

# JOCK ITCH

Jock itch isn't just embarrassingly itchy; it can also be painful and is highly contagious. Luckily, aromatherapy treatments are usually able to make short work of the *Tinea cruris* fungus, which causes this issue.

## Tea Tree-Citronella Balm

Makes about 2 ounces

Tea tree and citronella essential oils are strong antifungal agents that also help stop itching and cool stinging.

1 tablespoon coconut oil, melted
1 tablespoon hemp oil
1 tablespoon shea butter
1 tablespoon sweet almond oil
40 drops tea tree essential oil
20 drops citronella essential oil

1. In a medium bowl, combine all the ingredients. Whisk to blend thoroughly, and then transfer the balm to a small jar.

2. With a cotton swab, apply a pea-size amount of the balm to each affected area. Use a new cotton swab for each affected area. Repeat the treatment two to three times daily, continuing for 1 week after jock itch disappears.

## Lemon-Clove Bud Spray

Makes about 8 ounces

Lemon and clove bud essential oils kill fungus while numbing the itch. Witch hazel and fractionated coconut oil bring additional relief.

6 ounces distilled water
1 ounce fractionated coconut oil
1 ounce witch hazel
40 drops clove bud essential oil
40 drops lemon essential oil

1. In a bottle with a fine-mist spray top, combine all the ingredients. Shake well to blend, and then shake again before each use.

2. Apply 1 spritz to each affected area. Use two to three times daily, continuing for 1 week after jock itch disappears.

PREFERENCE TIP If you prefer, you can use this mixture as a toner by applying it with a cotton ball. To prevent cross-contamination, use a new cotton ball for each affected area.

## Geranium-Lemongrass Gel

Makes about 4 ounces

Geranium and lemongrass are an excellent combination for stopping the itch and killing fungus. Aloe vera gel provides comfort and promotes healing.

3½ ounces aloe vera gel
1 tablespoon fractionated coconut oil
40 drops geranium essential oil
40 drops lemongrass essential oil

1. In a large bowl, combine all the ingredients. Whisk to blend thoroughly, and then transfer the gel to a jar.

2. Apply 1 teaspoon of the blend to the affected area, using a little more or less as needed. Repeat two to three times daily, continuing for 1 week after jock itch disappears.

STORAGE If you like, you can keep this gel in the refrigerator for an intense cooling sensation upon application; otherwise, keep in a cool, dark place.

# JOINT PAIN

Many conditions can cause joint pain. Once your doctor has determined the cause, you can use aromatherapy treatments alone or alongside medication, physical therapy, and other physician-recommended remedies.

## Peppermint-Pine Liniment

Makes about 4 ounces

Brisk peppermint and pine essential oils combine with soothing chamomile to penetrate deep into tissue, targeting inflammation while encouraging tight, stiff joints to relax.

2 ounces aloe vera gel
1 ounce fractionated coconut oil
1 ounce rubbing alcohol
40 drops peppermint essential oil
20 drops German or Roman chamomile essential oil
20 drops pine essential oil

1. In a large bowl, combine all the ingredients. Whisk to blend thoroughly, and then transfer the liniment to a jar.
2. Apply 1 teaspoon of the liniment to the affected area, using a little more or less as needed. Repeat two to three times daily while joint pain persists.

## Spruce Compress

Makes 1 treatment

Fragrant spruce essential oil is a potent anti-inflammatory agent with cortisone-like effects. When combined with soothing heat, it eases pain quickly.

6 drops fractionated coconut oil
6 drops spruce essential oil

1. In the palm of your hand, combine the ingredients.
2. Apply the blend to the affected joint, and massage the area, using small circular motions.
3. Sit or lie down and cover the affected joint with a warm heating pad, following the manufacturer's instructions for safe use. Leave the heating pad in place for at least 15 minutes. Repeat two to three times daily while pain persists.

## Benzoin Balm

Makes about 2 ounces

Benzoin essential oil increases circulation and gently warms tissue, helping ease pain and promote healing.

2 tablespoons shea butter
1 tablespoon coconut oil, melted
1 tablespoon hemp oil ·
40 drops benzoin essential oil

1. In a medium bowl, combine all the ingredients. Whisk to blend thoroughly, and then transfer the balm to a small jar.
2. Apply ½ teaspoon of balm to the affected joint, and massage the area, using light pressure and circular motions. Use a little more or less of the balm as needed to cover the painful area, and repeat as often as needed to keep pain to a minimum.

# MENOPAUSE

Although it can be uncomfortable, menopause is a normal part of the aging process. Aromatherapy can help with hot flashes, irritability, disrupted sleep, and other symptoms by stimulating the endocrine system and balancing hormones, plus it can soothe specific symptoms.

## Peppermint-Rose Geranium Gel for Hot Flashes

Makes about 4 ounces

Crisp peppermint combines with fragrant rose geranium essential oil to provide relief from hot flashes. Aloe vera gel provides an additional cooling sensation as it is absorbed by the skin.

3½ ounces aloe vera gel
1 tablespoon fractionated coconut oil
40 drops rose geranium essential oil
20 drops peppermint essential oil

1. In a large bowl, combine all the ingredients. Whisk to blend thoroughly, and then transfer the gel to a jar.

2. Apply a dime-size amount of the blend to the back of your neck when you feel a hot flash coming. Use a little more or less as needed, and repeat as needed throughout the day.

STORAGE If you like, you can keep this gel in the refrigerator for an intense cooling sensation upon application; otherwise, keep in a convenient location.

## Balancing Vitex Berry Lotion

Makes about 8 ounces

Vitex berry reduces the levels of estrogen and increases the levels of progesterone, while rose and May Chang lift the spirits and offer an irresistible fragrance. Vitex berry takes at least two months to make a real impact, so be sure to use this lotion daily.

8 ounces unscented body lotion
   or hand cream
64 drops vitex berry essential oil
40 drops May Chang essential oil
40 drops pre-diluted rose oil
   or 4 drops rose otto

1. In a large bowl, combine all the ingredients. Whisk to blend thoroughly, and then transfer the lotion to a jar or back to its original container.

2. Apply 1 teaspoon of the blend to your wrists and inner arms. Use a little more or less as needed, and feel free to apply the lotion to other body parts. Use twice daily.

STORAGE Keep this lotion in a convenient location if you plan to use it all within two weeks; otherwise, keep it in a glass bottle or jar in a cool, dark place.

## Clary Sage Shower Melts

Makes 24 treatments

Comforting clary sage, geranium, and Roman chamomile combine with lavender and the steam from your shower to provide deep relaxation and relieve menopause symptoms.

5 cups baking soda
1 cup water
48 drops clary sage essential oil
24 drops geranium essential oil
24 drops lavender essential oil
24 drops Roman chamomile essential oil

1. Preheat the oven to 350°F, and line muffin tins with 24 cupcake liners.

2. In a large bowl, combine baking soda and water. Stir into a thick paste.

3. Evenly divide the paste between the cupcake liners, and bake for 20 minutes or until dry.

4. Allow the melts to cool completely, and then peel the liners off. To each melt, add 2 drops of clary sage, 1 drop of geranium, 1 drop of lavender essential oil, and 1 drop of Roman chamomile to each melt. Transfer the melts immediately to a wide-mouth jar or storage container.

5. Place 1 melt in the shower stall just before stepping in. Breathe deeply while you enjoy the fragrant steam. Repeat each evening to minimize nighttime menopause symptoms.

# MENSTRUAL SYMPTOMS

As if PMS isn't bad enough, menstruation comes with its own set of complications. Cramping, bloating, and irregularity are a few of the most common. Remember to check in with your doctor at least once a year to ensure that your menstrual symptoms are not a sign of an underlying medical problem.

## Cypress-German Chamomile Compress for Menstrual Cramps

Makes 1 treatment

Uplifting cypress and soothing German chamomile combine with heat to relax uterine muscle tissue and provide you with an emotional boost.

½ teaspoon fractionated coconut oil
5 drops cypress essential oil
5 drops geranium essential oil

1. In the palm of your hand, combine all the ingredients.
2. Apply the blend to your lower abdomen, targeting the uterine area, and gently massage the blend in.
3. Lie down and cover your lower abdomen with a hot heating pad, following the manufacturer's instructions for safe use. Leave the heating pad in place for at least 15 minutes. Repeat two to three times daily while suffering from cramps.

PREFERENCE TIP If you'd like to use this compress at bedtime, add 2 to 4 drops of lavender essential oil to the blend for extra relaxation.

## Fennel Seed-Grapefruit Massage for Bloating

Makes about 4 ounces

Soothing fennel seed and grapefruit essential oils increase circulation and encourage the body to release excess water, helping ease uncomfortable bloating.

2 tablespoons coconut oil, melted
2 tablespoons hemp oil
2 tablespoons shea butter
2 tablespoons sweet almond oil
64 drops grapefruit essential oil
32 drops fennel seed essential oil

1. In a medium bowl, combine all the ingredients. Whisk to blend thoroughly, and then transfer the message oil to a small jar.

2. Apply 1 teaspoon of the blend to the abdomen, and massage the area, using light, gentle strokes. Apply 1 more teaspoon of the blend to your lower back, just above the buttocks, and massage in. Repeat two to three times daily until menstrual bloating subsides.

## Synergistic Blend for Irregular Cycles

Makes about 4 ounces

A combination of Roman chamomile, geranium, fennel seed, vitex berry, and clary sage helps balance hormones and promotes regular menstruation. This blend often takes up to two months to start working, so be sure to use it daily.

4 ounces sweet almond oil
60 drops clary sage essential oil
60 drops Roman chamomile essential oil
60 drops vitex berry essential oil
44 drops geranium essential oil
22 drops fennel seed essential oil

1. In a bottle or jar, combine all the ingredients. Shake to blend.

2. Apply 1 drop of the blend to the inside of each elbow, and repeat twice daily.

# MIGRAINE

Migraines can sideline you, turning even the simplest tasks into major undertakings. Instead of reaching for strong pharmaceuticals when you feel a migraine coming on, give aromatherapy a try. If you have painful headaches frequently, be sure to have your doctor rule out a serious underlying condition.

## Palo Santo-Peppermint Balm

Makes about 4 ounces

Fragrant palo santo, frankincense, and peppermint combine to ease pain, increase circulation, and reduce the stress of a migraine.

3½ ounces aloe vera gel
1 tablespoon fractionated coconut oil
20 drops frankincense essential oil
20 drops palo santo essential oil
16 drops peppermint essential oil

1. In a large bowl, combine all the ingredients. Whisk to blend thoroughly, and then transfer the balm to a jar.

2. Apply 1 teaspoon of the blend to the back of your neck, and lightly massage the area. If pain is radiating from a certain part of your head, apply 1 drop of the blend to that spot, as well, and massage in. Repeat every 2 to 3 hours.

STORAGE If you like, you can keep this gel in the refrigerator for an intense cooling sensation upon application; otherwise, keep in a cool, dark place.

## Synergistic Migraine Blend

Makes 100 treatments

Bergamot, grapefruit, rosemary, peppermint, and Roman chamomile combine with lavender ease stress, promote relaxation, and help reduce the feelings of nausea that often accompany migraines.

2 teaspoons sweet almond oil
1 teaspoon lavender essential oil
20 drops grapefruit essential oil
20 drops petitgrain essential oil
12 drops Roman chamomile essential oil
8 drops peppermint essential oil
8 drops rosemary essential oil

1. In a small bottle, preferably with a roll-on applicator, combine all the ingredients. Shake well to blend.

2. With your fingertips or the roller, apply 1 drop of the blend to the bridge of your nose, and 1 drop to each of your temples. Apply 3 to 4 more drops of the blend to the base of your skull.

3. Massage each area lightly, and then apply a towel-wrapped ice pack to the back of your neck while you lie on your back for 15 minutes. Repeat two to three times daily as needed.

STORAGE Keep in a convenient location if you plan to use it up within a few weeks; otherwise, keep in a cool, dark place for up to a year.

## Synergistic Migraine Bath Salts

Makes 8 treatments

Roman chamomile, lavender, rosemary, peppermint, and clary sage essential oils combine with Epsom salt to ease pain, increase circulation, and help you relax. This treatment promotes restful sleep and is best for bedtime use.

2 tablespoons fractionated coconut oil
24 drops clary sage essential oil
24 drops lavender essential oil
16 drops Roman chamomile essential oil
8 drops peppermint essential oil
8 drops rosemary essential oil
4 cups Epsom salt

1. In a large bowl, combine the fractionated coconut oil and the essential oils. Add the Epsom salt and stir well to blend. Transfer the bath salts to a jar.

2. Draw a hot bath and add ½ cup of bath salts. Soak in the bath for at least 15 minutes. Repeat once daily whenever a migraine is present.

# MOODINESS

Discomfort, disease, medication side effects, or plain old bad days are among the causes of moodiness. If you are frequently irritable, have your doctor check for underlying illness; in the meantime, try these uplifting aromatherapy treatments.

## Tangerine-Lavender Lotion
Makes about 8 ounces

Cheery tangerine and relaxing lavender essential oils combine to alter your mental state so that you feel a bit less cranky.

8 ounces unscented body lotion
   or hand cream
30 drops tangerine essential oil
20 drops lavender essential oil

1. In a large bowl, combine all the ingredients. Whisk to blend thoroughly, and then transfer the lotion to a jar or back to its original container.

2. Apply 1 teaspoon of the blend to your hands, arms, and shoulders. Use a little more or less as needed, and feel free to apply the lotion to other body parts. Use as often as you like throughout each day, especially after washing your hands.

STORAGE Keep this lotion in a convenient location if you plan to use it all within two weeks; otherwise, keep it in a glass bottle or jar in a cool, dark place.

## Lemon, Rosemary, and Chamomile Diffusion

Makes 1 treatment

When stress and overwork are part of the equation, lemon, rosemary, and chamomile essential oils can perk you up, help you focus, and provide you with a bit more balance.

3 drops lemon essential oil
1 drop Roman or German chamomile essential oil
1 drop rosemary essential oil

Add the essential oils to your diffuser according to the manufacturer's instructions. Run the diffuser nearby.

SUBSTITUTION TIP If you need to go to sleep within four hours of using this diffusion blend, swap out the rosemary, which promotes alertness that can last for hours, for 1 drop of lavender.

## Sandalwood-Mandarin Spray

Makes about 8 ounces

Sandalwood and mandarin lift your spirits quickly while promoting a sense of peaceful awareness. If you tend to feel extra-annoyed while driving in traffic, this is a great blend to try because it won't make you sleepy. This blend smells so delicious that you might adopt it as your personal fragrance.

7 ounces distilled water
1 ounce witch hazel
30 drops sandalwood essential oil
20 drops mandarin essential oil

1. In a bottle with a fine-mist spray top, combine all the ingredients. Shake well to blend, and then shake again before each use.

2. Apply 1 spritz to each of the pulse points behind your ears, your inner elbows, and your wrists. You can also spritz clothing, your hair, or the air around you. Repeat as needed.

# MORNING SICKNESS

With persistent nausea and vomiting that tends to be at its worst in the morning, morning sickness can make you dread daybreak. You might also find that you are extra-sensitive to odors. Aromatherapy is among the best ways to rid yourself of these queasy feelings so you can enjoy your pregnancy more fully.

## Spearmint Pillowcase

Makes 1 treatment

Like its stronger cousin, peppermint, spearmint offers relief from nausea. This treatment works best when you use it every night.

**1 drop spearmint essential oil**

Just before lying down for the evening, apply the spearmint essential oil to your pillowcase. Breathe deeply as you relax. Repeat nightly.

## Fennel Seed Vapor

Makes 1 treatment

Fennel seed calms your stomach quickly while helping block out odors that bring on feelings of nausea.

1 cup steaming hot water
1 drop fennel seed essential oil

1. Pour the water into a large mug, and then add the essential oil.
2. Hold the mug in front of you and breathe in the vapors as you relax. Continue until the water cools. Repeat up to three times daily while morning sickness is present.

## Lavender-Lemon Inhaler

Makes 1 reusable inhaler

Lavender and lemon essential oils smell incredible together; they also calm the nervous system to help prevent nausea and vomiting while giving your mood a boost.

12 drops lavender essential oil
3 drops lemon essential oil

1. In a small bottle, combine the ingredients. Shake well to blend.
2. Apply the blend to the cotton wick of the aromatherapy inhaler.
3. Hold the inhaler beneath your nose, and inhale slowly through both nostrils to a count of five. Hold your breath for another count of five, and then exhale slowly. Repeat as needed to prevent and soothe symptoms.

SUBSTITUTION TIP If you don't have an inhaler, you can transfer the blend to a small, dark glass bottle and inhale directly from the bottle, or place 3 drops of the blend in your diffuser.

# MOTION SICKNESS

Queasiness and vomiting make motion sickness unbearable for the sufferer and unpleasant for fellow travelers, as well. Because it can be difficult to stop motion sickness symptoms once they begin, it's best to start using these treatments before movement takes place, and to continue using them throughout your journey.

## Ginger Inhaler

Makes 1 reusable inhaler

Ginger is such a reliable remedy for motion sickness that it is often called the traveler's friend. This inhaler makes it quick and easy to prevent symptoms on the road and in the air.

**12 drops ginger essential oil**

1. Apply the essential oil to the wick of an aromatherapy inhaler.

2. Hold the inhaler beneath your nose, and inhale slowly through both nostrils to a count of five. Hold your breath for another count of five, and then exhale slowly. Do this six to seven times every 30 minutes or so, beginning an hour before you set off on your journey. Repeat as needed to prevent and soothe symptoms.

SUBSTITUTION TIP If you don't have an inhaler, you can put the ginger in a small, dark glass bottle and inhale directly from the bottle, or place 3 drops of the ginger essential oil in your diffuser.

## Peppermint-Basil Travel Gel

Makes about 4 ounces

If you tend to sweat and feel nauseated while traveling, peppermint, basil, and lavender can help by calming smooth muscle tissues and cooling the heat.

3½ ounces aloe vera gel
1 tablespoon fractionated coconut oil
20 drops lavender essential oil
20 drops peppermint essential oil
12 drops basil essential oil

1. In a large bowl, combine all the ingredients. Whisk to blend thoroughly, and then transfer the gel to a jar.

2. Apply ½ teaspoon of the gel to the back of your neck about 30 minutes before setting out on your travels. Reapply every hour or so during travel.

## Synergistic Traveler's Body Lotion

Makes about 8 ounces

Roman chamomile, ginger, peppermint, and lemon combine to quell nausea and keep you in a positive mood as you travel.

8 ounces unscented body lotion
    or hand cream
30 drops ginger essential oil
20 drops lemon essential oil
10 drops peppermint essential oil
10 drops Roman chamomile essential oil

1. In a large bowl, combine all the ingredients. Whisk to blend thoroughly, and then transfer the lotion to a jar or back to its original container.

2. Apply 1 teaspoon of the lotion to your hands, arms, neck, and shoulders about 30 minutes before setting out. Use a little more or less as needed, and feel free to apply the lotion to other body parts. Apply another ½ teaspoon or so hourly while traveling, targeting your hands and the back of your neck.

STORAGE Keep this lotion in a convenient location if you plan to use it all within two weeks; otherwise, keep it in a glass bottle or jar in a cool, dark place.

# MUSCLE CRAMPS

Cramps occur when muscles tighten involuntarily. Depleted mineral levels, dehydration, overexercise, and nerve irritation are some causes, so be sure to address them while using aromatherapy treatments to bring relief.

## Soothing Massage Oil

Makes 1 ounce

Ginger, cinnamon leaf, and black pepper warm muscle fibers and encourage them to relax while simultaneously helping you to feel less stressed.

1 ounce fractionated coconut oil
4 drops black pepper essential oil
4 drops cinnamon leaf essential oil
2 drops ginger essential oil

1. In a small bottle or jar, combine all the ingredients. Shake well to blend.

2. Apply ½ teaspoon of the blend to the area where cramping is present, and massage in, using deep, firm strokes. Repeat two to three times daily or as needed.

## Lavender-Marjoram Compress

Makes 1 treatment

Lavender and marjoram combine with soothing heat to promote relaxation while easing the pain that accompanies cramping.

½ teaspoon fractionated coconut oil
3 drops lavender essential oil
2 drops marjoram essential oil

1. In the palm of your hand, combine all the ingredients.

2. Apply the blend to the cramped muscle, and massage in, using deep, firm strokes.

3. Sit or lie down comfortably, and cover the cramped muscle with a warm heating pad, following the manufacturer's instructions for safe use. Leave the heating pad in place for at least 15 minutes. Repeat two to three times daily or as needed.

## Minty Lavender-Cypress Gel

Makes about 4 ounces

Peppermint, lavender, and cypress essential oils come together to ease inflammation and help relax tight, cramping muscles.

3½ ounces aloe vera gel
1 tablespoon fractionated coconut oil
20 drops peppermint essential oil
16 drops cypress essential oil
12 drops lavender essential oil

1. In a large bowl, combine all the ingredients. Whisk to blend thoroughly, and then transfer the gel to a jar.

2. Apply 1 teaspoon of the gel to the affected area, using a little more or less as needed. Repeat two to three times daily or as needed.

STORAGE If you like, you can keep this gel in the refrigerator for an intense cooling sensation upon application; otherwise, keep in a cool, dark place.

# MUSCLE SORENESS

Repetitive or strenuous activity often leads to sore muscles. The discomfort may make you want to reach for an over-the-counter pain reliever, but give aromatherapy a try instead.

## Benzoin-Black Pepper Muscle Balm

Makes about 4 ounces

Benzoin and black pepper increase circulation and provide a warming sensation, helping ease your discomfort so that you can rest or get on with your day.

1 ounce beeswax, melted
1 ounce coconut oil, melted
1 ounce shea butter
1 tablespoon avocado oil
1 tablespoon sweet almond oil
40 drops benzoin essential oil
20 drops black pepper essential oil

1. In a medium bowl, combine all the ingredients. Whisk to blend thoroughly, and then transfer the balm to a small jar.

2. Apply 1 teaspoon of balm to the sore area, using a little more or less as needed. Repeat every 2 to 3 hours to stay comfortable until recovered.

## Synergistic Pain-Relief Compress

Makes 1 treatment

Warm ginger, cinnamon leaf, and cajuput combine with comforting German chamomile and soothing heat to provide deep, penetrating relief for sore muscles.

1 teaspoon avocado oil
4 drops cinnamon leaf essential oil
3 drops cajuput essential oil
3 drops German chamomile essential oil
2 drops ginger essential oil

1. In the palm of your hand, combine all the ingredients.

2. Apply the blend to the sore area, and massage in. (For a larger area, double or triple the ingredients, and combine them in a jar.)

3. Relax and cover the sore area with a warm heating pad, following the manufacturer's instructions for safe use. Leave the heating pad in place for at least 15 minutes. Repeat once or twice daily until recovered.

## Fir Needle Gel

Makes about 4 ounces

Fir needle stops muscle pain quickly, and its bright, uplifting aroma helps you deal with any accompanying mental fatigue.

3½ ounces aloe vera gel
40 drops fir needle essential oil

1. In a large bowl, combine the ingredients. Whisk to blend thoroughly, and then transfer the gel to a jar.

2. Apply 1 teaspoon of the gel to the affected area, using a little more or less as needed. Repeat two to three times daily.

STORAGE If you like, you can keep this gel in the refrigerator for an intense cooling sensation upon application; otherwise, keep in a cool, dark place.

# MUSCLE SPASMS/ RESTLESS LEGS SYNDROME

While muscle spasms aren't painful, they can be distressing. If you suffer from restless legs syndrome, it can seem impossible to get to sleep. Aromatherapy treatments can help stop the spasms by relaxing the muscles. If spasms happen frequently, check in with your doctor to rule out any underlying medical cause.

## Synergistic Muscle Spasm Blend

Makes 1 ounce

Cypress and ginger combine with marjoram essential oil, delivering deep, penetrating warmth that relieves tight, tense feelings and encourages muscle tissue to relax.

**1 ounce fractionated coconut oil**
**4 drops cypress essential oil**
**4 drops marjoram essential oil**
**2 drops ginger essential oil**

1. In a small bottle or jar, combine all the ingredients. Shake well to blend.
2. Apply ½ teaspoon to the area where spasms are present, and lightly massage the area. Repeat two to three times daily or as needed.

## Synergistic Muscle Spasm Compress

Makes 1 treatment

Marjoram, juniper, and basil essential oils work wonders to stop muscle spasms, and when soothing heat is added to the mix, the relaxing effect is intensified.

½ teaspoon fractionated coconut oil
1 drop basil essential oil
1 drop juniper essential oil
1 drop marjoram essential oil

1. In the palm of your hand, combine all the ingredients.

2. Apply the blend to the spasm site, and massage the area.

3. Sit or lie down and cover the area with a warm heating pad, following the manufacturer's instructions for safe use. Leave the heating pad in place for at least 15 minutes. Repeat two to three times daily or as needed.

## Lavender-Basil Bath Salts for Restless Legs Syndrome

Makes 8 treatments

A warm Epsom salt bath spiked with soothing lavender and basil essential oils help stop spasms, so you can relax and get that good night's rest you've been wanting.

2 tablespoons fractionated coconut oil
24 drops lavender essential oil
8 drops basil essential oil
4 cups Epsom salt

1. In a large bowl, combine the fractionated coconut oil and the essential oils. Add the Epsom salt and stir well to blend. Transfer the bath salts to a jar.

2. Draw a hot bath and add ½ cup of bath salts. Soak in the bath for at least 15 minutes. Repeat once daily while suffering from restless legs syndrome.

# NAUSEA/ VOMITING

Certain medications, over-consumption of alcohol, and cancer treatments are just a few of the things that can cause nausea and/or vomiting. If you suffer from frequent nausea and haven't identified the cause, see your doctor to rule out a serious underlying illness. Aromatherapy can help reduce or eliminate symptoms in the meantime.

## Melissa-Spearmint Bath Salts

Makes 8 treatments

Melissa and spearmint essential oils offer antispasmodic action and calm nerves, helping with both the physical and emotional distress that accompanies nausea.

2 tablespoons sweet almond oil
24 drops melissa essential oil
4 drops spearmint essential oil
4 cups Epsom salt

1. In a large bowl, combine the almond oil and the essential oils. Add the Epsom salt and stir well to blend. Transfer the bath salts to a jar.

2. Draw a warm bath and add ½ cup of bath salts. Soak in the bath for at least 15 minutes. Repeat once daily or as needed.

## Soothing Sandalwood Lotion

Makes about 8 ounces

Sandalwood smells fantastic and is great for skin, plus it helps put a stop to nausea while relieving stress. Sandalwood also helps the body detoxify itself, so if dietary indiscretion is behind your discomfort, this is a good remedy to try.

8 ounces unscented body lotion
or hand cream
20 drops sandalwood essential oil

1. In a large bowl, combine all the ingredients. Whisk to blend thoroughly, and then transfer the lotion to a jar or back to its original container.

2. Apply 1 teaspoon of the blend to your hands, arms, and shoulders. Use a little more or less as needed, and feel free to apply the lotion to other body parts. Use as often as you like.

STORAGE Keep this lotion in a convenient location if you plan to use it all within two weeks; otherwise, keep it in a glass bottle or jar in a cool, dark place.

## Copaiba-Chamomile Compress

Makes 1 treatment

Copaiba and German chamomile combine with soothing heat to stop stomach spasms and help you relax in the midst of your malady.

½ teaspoon fractionated coconut oil
2 drops copaiba essential oil
2 drops German chamomile essential oil

1. In the palm of your hand, combine all the ingredients.

2. Apply the blend to your upper abdomen, and gently massage the area in a clockwise direction.

3. Lie down and cover your upper abdomen with a warm heating pad, following the manufacturer's instructions for safe use. Leave the heating pad in place for at least 15 minutes. Repeat two to three times daily while suffering from nausea.

# NECK PAIN

Stress, poor ergonomics, and muscle strain are among the chief causes of neck pain. Aromatherapy treatments offer quick, nontoxic relief by reducing inflammation, promoting relaxation, and dissipating stress.

## Juniper-Peppermint Gel
Makes about 4 ounces

Juniper berry and peppermint essential oils stop pain quickly while targeting inflammation and helping dispel unpleasant emotions such as stress and anxiety.

3½ ounces aloe vera gel
1 tablespoon fractionated coconut oil
20 drops juniper berry essential oil
20 drops peppermint essential oil

1. In a large bowl, combine all the ingredients. Whisk to blend thoroughly, and then transfer the gel to a jar.

2. Apply ½ teaspoon of the blend to the back of your neck, and massage the area, using deep up-and-down strokes. Repeat two to three times daily.

STORAGE If you like, you can keep this gel in the refrigerator for an intense cooling sensation upon application; otherwise, keep in a cool, dark place.

## Marjoram-Fir Needle Compress

Makes 1 treatment

Relaxing marjoram and fir needle combine with heat to increase circulation, soothe spasms, and stop pain quickly. The uplifting fragrance helps with stress, too.

½ teaspoon fractionated coconut oil
1 drop fir needle essential oil
1 drop marjoram essential oil

1. In the palm of your hand, combine all the ingredients.
2. Apply the blend to the back of your neck, and gently massage the area.
3. Sit or lie down and cover your neck area with a warm heating pad, following the manufacturer's instructions for safe use. Leave the heating pad in place for at least 15 minutes. Repeat two to three times daily or as needed.

## Synergistic Pain-Relief Blend

Makes about 12 treatments

Warming basil, cool peppermint, lavender, cypress, and marjoram combine to increase blood flow and stop pain while targeting stress, muscle tension, spasms, and cramping.

1 ounce sweet almond oil
12 drops cypress essential oil
12 drops lavender essential oil
6 drops basil essential oil
6 drops marjoram essential oil
6 drops peppermint essential oil

1. In a small bottle or jar, combine all the ingredients. Shake well to blend.
2. With your fingers, apply ½ teaspoon of the blend to the base of your skull and the back and sides of your neck. Massage the area, using deep, kneading motions. Repeat every 2 to 3 hours or as often as needed.

# NERVOUSNESS

Nervousness is a state of hyper-awareness that keeps us physically and emotionally on edge. Whether you're chronically nervous or simply suffer from edginess before important events, aromatherapy can help ease the jitters and help you see things in a more positive light.

## Patchouli-Petitgrain Spritz

Makes about 8 ounces

Petitgrain and patchouli promote a sense of calm self-awareness while giving your mood a wonderful boost. You can use this spray on your skin, hair, and clothing, and even as an air freshener.

7 ounces distilled water
1 ounce witch hazel
14 drops patchouli essential oil
10 drops petitgrain essential oil

1. In a bottle with a fine-mist spray top, combine all the ingredients. Shake well to blend, and then shake again before each use.

2. Apply 1 spritz to your pulse points, targeting the areas behind your ears, on your inner wrists, and in the bend of each elbow. Repeat as needed to take the edge off.

## Clary Sage-Citrus Diffusion

Makes 1 treatment

Clary sage and cheerful citrus essential oils combine with a touch of jasmine to calm your nerves and ground your emotions.

2 drops clary sage essential oil
2 drops pre-diluted jasmine essential oil
1 drop lemon essential oil
1 drop mandarin essential oil

Add the essential oils to your diffuser according to the manufacturer's instructions. Run the diffuser nearby. Repeat every 2 to 3 hours or as needed.

## Calming Chamomile-Neroli Steam

Makes 1 treatment

Fragrant neroli and soothing Roman chamomile combine with the steam from your shower to deliver a heavenly fragrance and help bring you peace of mind.

6 drops Roman chamomile essential oil
3 drops neroli essential oil

1. Apply the essential oils to a folded washcloth and position it on the shower floor, opposite the area where you stand.

2. Enjoy a hot, steamy shower and breathe deep while relaxing and dwelling on positive thoughts. Repeat once or twice daily while dealing with nervousness.

# NOSEBLEED

Dry air and trauma are two main contributors to nosebleed. As long as your nose hasn't been broken, aromatherapy can help. If you have chronic nosebleeds, consult with your doctor to rule out an underlying cause.

## Cypress Nasal Compress

Makes 1 treatment

Cypress essential oil is a vasoconstrictor, meaning that it narrows blood vessels. This narrowing effect helps stop a nosebleed.

**1 drop cypress essential oil**

1. On a facial tissue, apply the cypress essential oil.

2. Lie down or tilt your head back, tuck the tissue into the affected nostril, and pinch your nostrils slightly together while breathing through your mouth. Leave the compress in place for 15 minutes, even if it seems like the bleeding has stopped.

## Lemon-Lavender Nasal Compress

Makes 1 treatment

Lemon essential oil is a hemostatic, meaning it encourages blood to clot faster. Lavender essential oil and an ice pack applied to the back of the neck soothe pain and encourage faster healing.

1 drop lemon essential oil
4 drops lavender essential oil

1. Moisten a cotton ball with 2 drops of water and add the lemon essential oil. Insert the cotton ball into the affected nostril.

2. Apply the lavender essential oil directly to the back of your neck.

3. Wrap an ice pack in a towel, and lie down with the ice pack under your neck. Rest for at least 15 minutes, and then remove the cotton ball. Repeat as needed.

## Lavender Nasal Salve

Makes 1 tablespoon

If your nosebleeds are occurring because of overexposure to dry air, this salve can help. Lavender heals the nasal lining, while coconut oil provides deep moisture where it's needed most.

1 tablespoon fractionated coconut oil
10 drops lavender essential oil

1. In a small bottle, combine the ingredients. Shake to blend.

2. With a cotton swab, apply 1 drop of the salve to the inner lining of the nose, focusing on the central portion that divides the nostrils. Repeat once or twice daily as long as dry air conditions are present.

# PINKEYE

Also known as conjunctivitis, pinkeye is normally caused by the same viruses that send colds, sore throats, and other illnesses around schools and communities. Aromatherapy treatments help ease the itch while helping stop the virus, without actually touching the eye.

## Synergistic Pinkeye Blend

Makes 1 tablespoon

Tea tree, lemon, frankincense, and cypress combine with other antiviral, antibacterial, and anti-inflammatory essential oils to stop pinkeye quickly. Do not attempt to apply the essential oils directly to eye tissue.

1 tablespoon fractionated coconut oil
9 drops lemon essential oil
9 drops tea tree essential oil
4 drops frankincense essential oil
4 drops helichrysum essential oil
4 drops lavender essential oil
2 drops cypress essential oil
2 drops *Eucalyptus globulus* essential oil
2 drops lemongrass essential oil

1. In a small bottle or jar, combine all the ingredients. Shake well to blend.

2. Carefully apply 1 drop of the blend to the top of the cheekbone, directly beneath the affected eye. Apply one more drop to the side of the nose, on the same side as the affected eye. Repeat two to three times daily until pinkeye is gone.

## Lavender-Tea Tree Compress

Makes 1 treatment

Lavender, tea tree, and *Eucalyptus globulus* essential oils offer a potent antibacterial effect when combined. Be very careful not to get any essential oil into the eye itself.

2 drops *Eucalyptus globulus* essential oil
1 drop lavender essential oil
1 drop tea tree essential oil

1. Fold a paper towel in quarters, and then apply the essential oils, one on top of the other.

2. Close the affected eye and place a cotton ball on the eyelid. Position the paper towel on top of the cotton ball.

3. Relax while holding the compress in place. Leave the treatment on the eye for 15 minutes, and then discard. Repeat two to three times daily until pinkeye is gone.

PREFERENCE TIP If you would rather not use the compress, blend the essential oils with 4 drops of carrier oil and apply the blend to the cheekbone and side of the nose.

## Cool Chamomile Compress

Makes 1 treatment

Chamomile offers antiseptic and anti-inflammatory action, but it is milder than other pinkeye treatments. If you feel a telltale itch in your eye but don't yet have full-blown conjunctivitis, this is a good remedy to try.

¼ cup distilled water
3 drops Roman or German chamomile

1. In a shallow bowl, combine the ingredients. Fold a washcloth lengthwise and use it to absorb the mixture from the bowl.

2. Wring out any excess moisture, and then lie down with your eyes closed. Lay the compress over both eyes and leave it in place for 15 minutes. Repeat two to three times daily until the itch is gone.

# POISON IVY

Poison ivy, as well as poison oak and poison sumac, contains a compound called urushiol, which causes a burning, blistered rash that spreads like wildfire if you scratch it. Aromatherapy treatments help, especially when combined with traditional remedies like calamine lotion, aloe vera gel, and baking soda.

## Lavender-Frankincense Bath

Makes 8 treatments

Lavender and frankincense essential oils combine with baking soda to soothe inflammation and stop itching. Follow up with Peppermint-Myrrh Lotion (page 191) or Synergistic Itch-Relief Spray (page 191) for even more relief.

**4 cups baking soda**
**24 drops lavender essential oil**
**16 drops frankincense essential oil**

1. In a large bowl, combine all the ingredients. Whisk to blend thoroughly, and then transfer the bath salts to a jar.

2. Draw a lukewarm bath and add 1/2 cup of bath salts. Soak in the bath for at least 15 minutes. Repeat once or twice daily until the rash is gone.

## Peppermint-Myrrh Lotion

Makes about 8 ounces

Soothing calamine lotion is a popular go-to when poison ivy strikes, but you can make it even more potent by adding peppermint and myrrh, both of which help relieve the itching.

8 ounces calamine lotion
40 drops peppermint essential oil
20 drops myrrh essential oil

1. In a large bowl, combine all the ingredients. Whisk to blend thoroughly, and then transfer the lotion to a jar.

2. Use a cotton ball to gently apply a pea-size amount of the blend to each affected area, working from the outer edge of the rash to the inside. Use a little more or less as needed, and prevent cross-contamination by using a new cotton ball to treat each affected area. Repeat every 2 hours until the rash is gone.

STORAGE Keep this lotion in a convenient location if you plan to use it all within two weeks; otherwise, keep it in a glass bottle or jar in a cool, dark place.

## Synergistic Itch-Relief Spray

Makes about 8 ounces

Lavender, helichrysum, geranium, cypress, chamomile, and peppermint essential oils combine with witch hazel and Epsom salt to deliver rapid relief from itching and burning.

4 ounces distilled water
4 ounces witch hazel
1 teaspoon Epsom salt
12 drops cypress essential oil
12 drops geranium essential oil
12 drops helichrysum essential oil
12 drops lavender essential oil
12 drops Roman chamomile essential oil
4 drops peppermint essential oil

1. In a bottle with a fine-mist spray top, combine all the ingredients. Shake very well to dissolve Epsom salt, and then shake again before each use.

2. Apply 1 spritz to each affected area. Repeat every 1 to 2 hours until the rash is gone.

# PREMENSTRUAL SYNDROME (PMS)

Moodiness, a sense of sadness, depression, and lower back pain are just a few of the symptoms that may accompany PMS. Aromatherapy treatments often work wonders, especially when you start using them at the first sign of symptoms.

## Bergamot-Rose Geranium Shower Melts

Makes 24 treatments

Bergamot, clary sage, and rose geranium help ease feelings of sadness, depression, and irritation associated with PMS, especially when combined with the steam from your hot shower.

5 cups baking soda
1 cup water
48 drops bergamot essential oil
48 drops clary sage essential oil
48 drops rose geranium essential oil

1. Preheat the oven to 350°F, and line a muffin tin with 24 cupcake liners.

2. In a small bowl, combine baking soda and water. Stir into a thick paste.

3. Evenly divide the paste between the cupcake liners, and bake for 20 minutes or until dry.

4. Allow the melts to cool completely, and then peel the liners off. To each melt, add 2 drops of each essential oil. Transfer the melts immediately to a wide-mouth jar or storage container.

5. Place 1 melt in the shower stall just before stepping in. Breathe deeply while you enjoy the fragrant steam. Repeat once or twice daily while battling PMS.

PREFERENCE TIP If you would rather enjoy a hot bath, just drop a melt into the water while you're filling the tub.

## Vetiver-Vitex Berry Balm

Makes 100 treatments

Vitex berry balances hormones and stops headaches so you feel less edgy, plus it helps put a stop to mood swings and food cravings. Vitex berry builds up slowly in the body, so you'll need to use it for at least two months before you begin to notice its effects. Vetiver and sandalwood boost your mood in the interim.

1 tablespoon sweet almond oil
24 drops vitex berry essential oil
12 drops sandalwood essential oil
8 drops vetiver essential oil

1. In a small bottle, preferably with a roll-on applicator, combine all the ingredients. Shake well to blend.

2. With your fingertips or the roller, apply 1 drop to the pulse point behind each of your ears, and gently massage the area. Repeat once daily.

STORAGE Keep in a convenient location if you plan to use it up within a few weeks; otherwise, keep in a cool, dark place for up to a year.

## Bergamot-Clary Sage Compress

Makes 1 treatment

Bergamot and clary sage combine with soothing heat to stop physical discomfort while bringing about a more positive state of mind.

½ teaspoon fractionated coconut oil
3 drops clary sage essential oil
1 drop bergamot essential oil

1. In the palm of your hand, combine all the ingredients.

2. Apply the blend to your lower back, and gently massage the area, focusing on the area just above your buttocks.

3. Lie down and cover your lower back with a warm heating pad, following the manufacturer's instructions for safe use. Leave the heating pad in place for at least 15 minutes. Repeat two to three times daily while suffering from PMS.

# PROSTATITIS

The average prostate gland is the size of a walnut; when prostatitis strikes, it can swell up to more than twice its normal size, squeezing the urethra and causing painful urination. If you think you have prostatitis, see your doctor immediately to rule out a more serious condition. Once you have received a diagnosis, you can use aromatherapy treatments alone or alongside other remedies.

## Myrrh Massage

Makes 1 treatment

Myrrh is a strong anti-inflammatory essential oil and is among the best for dealing with prostatitis. Because it can cause sensitive skin in some individuals, be sure to conduct a patch test before using this treatment on delicate areas.

**3 drops fractionated coconut oil**
**3 drops myrrh essential oil**

1. In the palm of your hand, combine the ingredients.
2. Apply the blend to the perineal area, which is located between the anus and scrotum. Repeat two to three times daily as needed.

## Synergistic Prostatitis Blend

Makes about 1 ounce

Thyme, lavender, cypress, and *Eucalyptus radiata* essential oils target pain and inflammation, easing swelling and addressing prostatitis symptoms.

1 ounce fractionated coconut oil
10 drops cypress essential oil
10 drops *Eucalyptus radiata* essential oil
5 drops lavender essential oil
5 drops thyme essential oil

1. In a small bottle or jar, combine all the ingredients. Shake well to blend.
2. Apply 1 teaspoon of the blend to the lower back and lower abdomen, and massage the area. Repeat twice daily.

## Frankincense-Myrrh Bath Salts

Makes 8 treatments

Frankincense, myrrh, and Spanish sage essential oils combine with Epsom salt to soothe inflammation, while hot water brings further relief from symptoms.

2 tablespoons fractionated coconut oil
24 drops myrrh essential oil
16 drops frankincense essential oil
6 drops Spanish sage essential oil
4 cups Epsom salt

1. In a large bowl, combine the fractionated coconut oil and the essential oils. Add the Epsom salt and stir well to blend. Transfer the bath salts to a jar.
2. Draw a hot bath and add ½ cup of bath salts. Soak in the bath for at least 15 minutes. Repeat once daily as long as discomfort persists.

# PSORIASIS

Psoriasis causes skin cells to grow about five times faster than normal, causing thick, flaking, itchy patches called *plaques*. Aromatherapy treatments don't cure psoriasis, but they provide relief from discomfort.

## Cajuput-Cucumber Seed Gel

Makes about 4 ounces

Refreshing cajuput and cucumber seed essential oils combine with cool aloe vera gel to soothe inflammation and stop itching.

3½ ounces aloe vera gel
1 tablespoon fractionated coconut oil
24 drops cucumber seed essential oil
12 drops cajuput essential oil

1. In a large bowl, combine all the ingredients. Whisk to blend thoroughly, and then transfer the gel to a jar.

2. Apply ½ teaspoon of the blend to the affected area, using a little more or less as needed. Repeat two to three times daily during flare-ups.

STORAGE  If you like, you can keep this gel in the refrigerator for an intense cooling sensation upon application; otherwise, keep in a cool, dark place.

## Helichrysum Spray

Makes about 8 ounces

Helichrysum essential oil is a potent anti-inflammatory, plus it helps damaged tissue repair itself quickly. If stress plays a part in your psoriasis, you'll appreciate its ability to promote relaxation, too.

4 ounces distilled water
4 ounces witch hazel
24 drops helichrysum essential oil

1. In a bottle with a fine-mist spray top, combine all the ingredients. Shake well to blend, and then shake again before each use.

2. Apply 1 spritz to each affected area. Repeat every 1 to 2 hours as needed.

## German Chamomile Bath Salts

Makes 8 treatments

Chamomile, bergamot, and lavender essential oils combine with Dead Sea salt and moisturizing fractionated coconut oil to soothe inflammation and stop itching.

3 tablespoons fractionated coconut oil
24 drops lavender essential oil
12 drops German chamomile essential oil
6 drops bergamot essential oil
4 cups Dead Sea salt
1 cup oat flour

1. In a large bowl, combine the fractionated coconut oil and the essential oils. Add the Dead Sea salt and stir well to blend. Add the oat flour and stir again until completely incorporated. Transfer the bath salts to a jar.

2. Draw a warm bath and add ½ cup of bath salts. Soak in the bath for at least 15 minutes. Repeat once or twice weekly while psoriasis is active.

# RELAXATION

Stress is linked to an enormous number of health problems, and taking time out to relax should be an important part of every day. Aromatherapy is an excellent tool for relaxation, and one that you'll eagerly look forward to using.

## Everyday Citrus-Sandalwood Spritzer

*Makes about 8 ounces*

Snappy citrus essential oils combine with sweet sandalwood to keep you, your car, and your home smelling fantastic while promoting a sense of calm relaxation. While most relaxation treatments help you unwind, this one promotes clarity. It's just right for spraying in your car before a stressful commute.

7 ounces distilled water
1 ounce witch hazel
10 drops sandalwood essential oil
10 drops sweet orange essential oil
5 drops grapefruit essential oil
5 drops lemon essential oil
5 drops lime essential oil

1. In a bottle with a fine-mist spray top, combine all the ingredients. Shake well to blend, and then shake again before each use.

2. Apply 3 to 4 spritzes on your body, your clothing, your car's upholstery, or the air in your home or office. Repeat as often as you like.

## Lavender-Chamomile Foot Lotion

Makes about 8 ounces

Lavender and Roman chamomile take the edge off perfectly, letting you unwind at the end of a stressful day. But make sure you're finished with important tasks before using this remedy.

8 ounces unscented body lotion
   or hand cream
28 drops Roman Chamomile essential oil
20 drops lavender essential oil

1. In a large bowl, combine all the ingredients. Whisk to blend thoroughly, and then transfer the lotion to a jar or back to its original container.

2. Apply 1 teaspoon of the blend to your feet, ankles, and lower legs. Use a little more or less as needed, and feel free to apply the lotion to other body parts. Repeat whenever you need to relax.

STORAGE Keep this lotion in a convenient location if you plan to use it all within two weeks; otherwise, keep it in a glass bottle or jar in a cool, dark place.

## Synergistic Relaxation Diffusion

Makes 40 to 50 treatments

Rosewood, lavender, chamomile, and geranium combine with ylang-ylang, clary sage, and marjoram to deliver an intoxicating aroma that promotes relaxation.

36 drops lavender essential oil
30 drops rosewood essential oil
24 drops geranium or rose geranium
   essential oil
24 drops Roman chamomile essential oil
20 drops clary sage essential oil
20 drops ylang-ylang essential oil
16 drops marjoram essential oil

1. In a small bottle, combine all the ingredients. Shake well to blend. With the cap secured, allow the different scents to marry for 24 to 48 hours before use.

2. Add 3 to 4 drops of the blend to your diffuser according to the manufacturer's instructions. Run the diffuser nearby. Repeat as often as you'd like to create a relaxing atmosphere in your home or office.

# RINGWORM

Circular, red lesions give ringworm its name, which leads some to believe that it's caused by a parasite. Instead, fungi called *dermatophytes* are to blame for this highly contagious rash. Aromatherapy treatments bring comfort and kill the fungus without causing unpleasant side effects.

## Tea Tree Neat Treatment for Severe Ringworm

Makes 1 treatment

Tea tree offers powerful antifungal properties; it's also among the few essential oils that can be placed on skin without a carrier oil. Be sure to conduct a patch test before using this neat treatment.

**1 drop tea tree essential oil**

1. With a cotton swab, apply 1 drop of tea tree essential oil to the affected area.

2. Repeat the treatment on all lesions, preventing cross-contamination by using a new cotton swab for each affected area. Repeat the treatment two to three times daily until ringworm is gone.

## Lavender Neat Treatment for Minor Ringworm

Makes 1 treatment

Lavender is an effective antifungal agent; it's also the mildest of all the essential oils that can be placed on skin without a carrier oil. Still, be sure to conduct a patch test before using this neat treatment.

1 drop lavender essential oil

1. With a cotton swab, apply 1 drop of lavender essential oil to the affected area as soon as you suspect ringworm is present.

2. Repeat the treatment on all potentially affected areas, preventing cross-contamination by using a new cotton swab for each affected area. Repeat the treatment two to three times daily until ringworm is gone.

## Synergistic Antifungal Spray

Makes about 8 ounces

Tea tree, lavender, myrrh, and lemongrass combine to create a potent antifungal spray that you can use when there are too many ringworm lesions to treat individually.

7 ounces organic apple cider vinegar
1 ounce fractionated coconut oil
40 drops lavender essential oil
40 drops tea tree essential oil
20 drops lemongrass essential oil
20 drops myrrh essential oil
10 drops peppermint essential oil

1. In a bottle with a fine-mist spray top, combine all the ingredients. Shake well to blend, and then shake again before each use.

2. Apply 1 spritz to each affected area two to three times daily until ringworm is gone.

# SHINGLES

The same virus that causes chicken pox is to blame for shingles, which appears as an angry, painful, blistered rash. Aromatherapy treatments can't cure shingles, but they can minimize pain and itching.

## Ravintsara Spray for Itchy or Painful Shingles

Makes about 4 ounces

Ravintsara essential oil is a powerful antiviral agent that also helps soothe pain and stop itching. It can cause sensitive skin in some individuals, so be sure to conduct a patch test before using this treatment.

**4 ounces witch hazel**
**40 drops ravintsara essential oil**

1. In a bottle with a fine-mist spray top, combine the ingredients. Shake well to blend, and then shake again before each use.

2. Apply 1 spritz to each affected area. Repeat every 2 to 3 hours as needed.

## Synergistic Gel
## for Painful Shingles

Makes about 4 ounces

Ravintsara, *Eucalyptus globulus*, and peppermint essential oils combine to stop pain and promote healing while attacking the shingles virus.

4 ounces aloe vera gel
40 drops *Eucalyptus globulus* essential oil
40 drops ravintsara essential oil
20 drops peppermint essential oil

1. In a large bowl, combine all the ingredients. Whisk to blend thoroughly, and then transfer the gel to a jar.

2. With a cotton swab, apply a pea-size amount of the blend to the affected area, using a little more or less as needed. Repeat twice daily during shingles flare-ups.

STORAGE If you like, you can keep this gel in the refrigerator for an intense cooling sensation upon application; otherwise, keep in a cool, dark place.

## Synergistic Blend
## for Emerging Shingles

Makes about 4 ounces

Helichrysum, ravintsara, lavender, peppermint, and *Eucalyptus globulus* essential oils combine with rosehip oil and fractionated coconut oil to moisturize skin while helping minimize shingles outbreaks.

3 ounces fractionated coconut oil
1 ounce rosehip oil
40 drops *Eucalyptus globulus* essential oil
40 drops helichrysum essential oil
40 drops lavender essential oil
40 drops ravintsara essential oil
20 drops peppermint essential oil

1. In a bottle or jar, combine all the ingredients. Shake well to blend.

2. At the first sign of discomfort, use a cotton swab to apply 2 drops of the blend to the site. Repeat each time you feel any itching or pain, and continue to apply to any rash that emerges until the episode ends.

STORAGE Carry the remedy with you as soon as shingles show signs of becoming active; otherwise, keep in a cool dark place.

# SINUSITIS

When sinuses become inflamed and irritated, chronic congestion and discomfort result. Aromatherapy addresses pain, congestion, inflammation, and infection, often eliminating the need for potentially toxic medicines. If pain worsens or symptoms persist despite your best efforts, see your doctor for something stronger.

## Synergistic Sinusitis Shower Melts

Makes 10 treatments

Eucalyptus, ginger, thyme, and tea tree essential oils combine with the steam from your hot shower to deliver quick relief from symptoms while addressing inflammation and targeting infection.

2 ½ cups baking soda
½ cup water
20 drops ginger essential oil
20 drops eucalyptus essential oil
20 drops thyme essential oil
20 drops tea tree essential oil

1. Preheat the oven to 350°F, and line a muffin tin with 10 cupcake liners.

2. In a small bowl, combine baking soda and water. Stir into a thick paste.

3. Evenly divide the paste between the cupcake liners, and bake for 20 minutes or until dry.

4. Allow the melts to cool completely, and then peel the liners off. To each melt, add 2 drops of each essential oil. Transfer the melts immediately to a wide-mouth jar or storage container.

5. Place 1 melt in the shower stall just before stepping in. Breathe deeply while you enjoy the fragrant steam. Repeat once or twice daily while sinusitis persists.

## Eucalyptus-Spearmint Vapor

Makes 1 treatment

Eucalyptus and spearmint essential oils work together to clear sinuses and kill bacteria, while warm steam moisturizes your sinuses.

2 cups steaming hot water
1 drop eucalyptus essential oil (any species)
1 drop spearmint essential oil

1. Pour the water into a large bowl, and then add the essential oils. Place a box of tissues nearby.

2. Sit comfortably in front of the bowl and drape a towel over your head and the bowl, creating a tent that concentrates the steam and vapors. Emerge to blow your nose or breathe cool air as needed. Try to spend 10 minutes with the treatment, and repeat it once or twice daily while you are recovering.

## Synergistic Sinusitis Inhaler

Makes 1 reusable inhaler

With this handy inhaler, eucalyptus, cedarwood, oregano, and niaouli essential oils combine to clear your sinuses and ease breathing whenever you take a sniff.

10 drops eucalyptus essential oil
5 drops cedarwood essential oil
5 drops oregano essential oil
3 drops niaouli essential oil

1. In a small bottle or jar, combine all essential oils. Shake well to blend.

2. Apply the blend to the cotton wick of the aromatherapy inhaler.

3. Hold the inhaler beneath your nose, and inhale slowly through both nostrils to a count of five. Hold your breath for another count of five, and then exhale slowly. Repeat as needed to prevent and soothe symptoms.

SUBSTITUTION TIP If you don't have an inhaler, you can transfer the blend to a small, dark glass bottle and inhale directly from the bottle, or place 3 drops of the blend in your diffuser.

# SKIN TAGS

Skin tags are benign lesions consisting of small flaps of tissues that hang from the skin via a slender connecting stalk. Your doctor can easily remove skin tags; however, you can use aromatherapy treatments to get rid of them yourself.

## Frankincense Neat Treatment

Makes 1 treatment

Frankincense essential oil shrinks skin tags by encouraging the tissue to dry up. If you get any pure frankincense essential oil on surrounding skin, dab a drop of carrier oil on it to prevent dryness. Be sure to conduct a patch test before using this neat treatment.

**1 drop frankincense essential oil**

1. With a cotton swab, apply the frankincense essential oil to the skin tag.

2. Repeat the treatment three times daily until the skin tag falls off. If your skin tag is very large, this may take up to three months.

## Oregano Neat Treatment

*Makes 1 treatment*

Oregano essential oil irritates skin tags and causes them to dry up quickly. This remedy stings, and you'll need to be sure to protect underlying skin. If the stinging is too intense, dilute the oregano oil with a drop of carrier oil before applying it to the skin tag.

2 drops carrier oil
1 drop oregano essential oil

1. With a cotton swab, carefully apply a layer of carrier oil to the skin beneath the skin tag.

2. With a fresh cotton swab, carefully apply the oregano essential oil to the skin tag. Repeat two to three times daily until the skin tag falls off. If your skin tag is very large, this may take up to 3 weeks.

## Tea Tree-Lemon Gel for Multiple Skin Tags

*Makes about 2 ounces*

Lemon and tea tree combine to dry up small skin tags without causing discomfort or burning underlying skin.

2 ounces aloe vera gel
40 drops lemon essential oil
40 drops tea tree essential oil

1. In a small bowl, combine all the ingredients. Whisk to blend thoroughly, and then transfer the gel to a jar.

2. With a cotton swab, apply 1 drop of the blend to the affected area, using a little more or less as needed. Repeat two to three times daily until skin tags are gone.

STORAGE If you like, you can keep this gel in the refrigerator for an intense cooling sensation upon application; otherwise, keep in a cool, dark place.

# SORE THROAT/ LARYNGITIS

A bacterial infection can leave you with a sore throat, and an evening spent cheering loudly for your favorite team can cause inflammation in your voice box, resulting in laryngitis. Whatever the case, aromatherapy helps by soothing pain and inflammation, and by targeting bacterial infections.

## Lavender-Marjoram Sore Throat Spray

Makes about 4 ounces

Soothing lavender and marjoram combine with sea salt to ease pain, minimize inflammation, and kill bacteria.

4 ounces warm water
½ teaspoon sea salt
4 drops marjoram essential oil
2 drops lavender essential oil

1. In a bottle with a fine-mist spray top, combine all the ingredients. Shake well to blend, and then shake again before each use.
2. Apply 2 to 3 spritzes to the back of your throat. Repeat hourly or as often as needed.

## Lavender-Lemon Gargle

Makes 8 ounces

Refreshing lemon and soothing lavender essential oils offer antiseptic and analgesic properties; they help bring comfort while killing bacteria and promoting healing.

7 ounces distilled water
1 ounce unflavored vodka
3 drops lemon essential oil
2 drops lavender essential oil

1. In a bottle or jar, combine all the ingredients. Shake well to blend, and then shake again before each use.

2. Pour 1 tablespoon of the blend into a glass, and then gargle for 30 seconds, being careful not to swallow. Spit out when finished. Repeat two to three times daily until recovered.

## Soothing Bergamot-Lavender Neck Wrap

Makes 1 treatment

Fragrant bergamot and lavender combine with potent tea tree essential oil to provide comfort while delivering a powerful antibacterial punch.

2 cups hot water
3 drops lavender essential oil
2 drops bergamot essential oil
1 drop tea tree essential oil

1. In a large bowl, combine all the ingredients. Soak a soft cloth in the water and wring it out.

2. Wrap the cloth securely around your neck and cover it with a second towel to hold the heat in. Remove the wrap before it cools completely. Repeat as often as you like.

# SPLINTER

Like paper cuts, tiny pieces of wood often cause an extraordinary amount of pain. Aromatherapy treatments help splinter sites heal quickly, plus they kill bacteria and ease discomfort.

## Lavender Neat Treatment

Makes 1 treatment

Lavender offers some pain relief while promoting faster healing. Its antibacterial property helps prevent infection. Be sure to conduct a patch test before using this neat treatment.

**1 drop lavender essential oil**

1. Wash the wound and gently pat it dry, and then use a sterilized needle or tweezer to remove the splinter.

2. Apply the lavender essential oil to the site by dripping it directly from the bottle, being careful not to touch the bottle to the splinter site. Repeat as often as needed for pain control.

## Soothing Helichrysum-Clove Bud Compress

Makes 1 treatment

Pain-relieving clove bud and soothing helichrysum combine with cold water to bring rapid relief and provide protection from infection.

**½ cup distilled water**
**2 ice cubes**
**1 drop clove bud essential oil**
**1 drop helichrysum essential oil**

1. Wash the wound and gently pat it dry, and then use a sterilized needle or tweezer to remove the splinter.

2. In a small bowl, pour the distilled water over the ice cubes, and then add the essential oils.

3. Soak a folded washcloth in the solution, and then place it on the sore spot. Top the washcloth with a folded hand towel to catch any drips.

4. Leave the compress in place for 10 to 15 minutes. Allow your skin to air-dry after removal, and repeat as needed to relieve pain.

## Elemi-Neroli First Aid Balm

Makes about 1 ounce

Fragrant neroli combines with antiseptic elemi to create a soothing first aid balm that stops pain quickly while helping prevent infection.

**1 ounce fractionated coconut oil**
**20 drops elemi essential oil**
**10 drops neroli essential oil**

1. In a small bottle or jar, combine all the ingredients. Shake well to blend.

2. Wash the wound and gently pat it dry, and then use a sterilized needle or tweezers to remove the splinter.

3. With a cotton swab, apply 1 to 2 drops of balm to the splinter site. Repeat as needed.

# SPRAIN

Painful, swollen ligament injuries occur when trauma causes a joint to move in a direction other than the one that it's meant to move. When combined with traditional first-aid measures including rest, ice compression, immobilization, and elevation, aromatherapy eases pain and helps you heal faster. Seek medical attention if you suspect you've broken a bone, or if swelling and pain fail to decrease after a day or two.

## Minty Helichrysum-Chamomile Compress

Makes 1 treatment

A soothing combination of peppermint, helichrysum, and chamomile essential oils brings quick pain relief and promotes healing, while a cold compress helps minimizing swelling.

4 drops helichrysum essential oil
2 drops carrier oil
2 drops German or Roman chamomile
2 drops peppermint essential oil

1. In the palm of your hand, combine all the ingredients.
2. Apply the blend to the sprain site, and gently massage the area. (Use another drop or two of each oil if you need to cover a large area.)
3. Wrap an ice pack in a hand towel, and then elevate the injury before laying the compress over the sprained area.
4. Leave the compress in place for 30 minutes, removing it periodically if your skin starts to feel uncomfortably numb. Repeat every hour or so during the first day to help the swelling come down.

## Synergistic First-Aid Gel and Sprain Compress

Makes about 4 ounces

Ginger, helichrysum, and lavender work together to stop pain and promote healing. On the first day of treatment, use this blend with an ice pack. Do not apply the heating pad on the first day of sprain treatment. On the second and third day, you can alternate between a heating pad and ice pack.

3½ ounces aloe vera gel
1 tablespoon fractionated coconut oil
36 drops lavender essential oil
24 drops helichrysum essential oil
12 drops ginger essential oil

1. In a large bowl, combine all the ingredients. Whisk to blend thoroughly, and then transfer the gel to a jar.

2. Apply 1 teaspoon of the gel to the affected area, using a little more or less as needed. Cover the area either with an ice pack or a warm heating pad, following the manufacturer's instructions for safe use. Leave the ice pack or heating pad in place for 15 to 20 minutes.

3. Reapply the gel each time you apply a heating pad or ice pack, ensuring that you keep the injury elevated as much as possible.

STORAGE If you like, you can keep this gel in the refrigerator for an intense cooling sensation upon application; otherwise, keep in a cool, dark place.

## Synergistic Healing Balm

Makes about 4 ounces

Lavender, marjoram, and peppermint help improve circulation while providing pain relief. This balm is ideal for application under compression bandages, as long as no broken skin is present.

2 ounces shea butter
1 ounce coconut oil, melted
1 ounce sweet almond oil
36 drops lavender essential oil
24 drops marjoram essential oil
12 drops peppermint essential oil

1. In a medium bowl, combine all the ingredients. Whisk to blend thoroughly, and then transfer the balm to a small jar.

2. Apply 1 teaspoon of balm to the sprain, using a little more or less as needed to cover as needed. Massage the balm in using light, gentle strokes, and then cover with a compression bandage. Repeat each time you re-bandage the sprain.

# STRESS

Often referred to as "the silent killer," stress is an uncomfortable state of emotional or mental strain that arises as the result of demanding or adverse circumstances. Aromatherapy treatments help ease the tension while you find healthy ways to decrease the amount of pressure in your life.

## Benzoin-Bergamot Lotion

Makes about 8 ounces

Benzoin and bergamot help your mind relax without making you feel sleepy, plus the blend is a fantastic one for keeping skin in good shape.

8 ounces unscented body lotion
  or hand cream
20 drops bergamot essential oil
10 drops benzoin essential oil

1. In a large bowl, combine all the ingredients. Whisk to blend thoroughly, and then transfer the lotion to a jar or back to its original container.

2. Apply 1 teaspoon of the lotion to your hands, arms, and shoulders. Use a little more or less as needed, and feel free to apply the lotion to other body parts. Use as often as you like throughout the day, especially after washing your hands.

STORAGE Keep this lotion in a convenient location if you plan to use it all within two weeks; otherwise, keep it in a glass bottle or jar in a cool, dark place.

## Cardamom-Mandarin Temple Rub

Makes 100 treatments

Warm, spicy cardamom blends with cheerful mandarin, uplifting your mood while alleviating stress. If you're feeling worried, depressed, or fatigued, this blend can help.

1 tablespoon sweet almond oil
20 drops mandarin essential oil
10 drops cardamom essential oil

1. In a small bottle, preferably with a roll-on applicator, combine all the ingredients. Shake well to blend.

2. With your fingertips or the roller, apply 1 drop to each of your temples, and then massage the areas gently while inhaling deeply.

PREFERENCE TIP If you like this fragrance and want to diffuse it, use a ratio of 1 drop of cardamom to 2 drops of mandarin to create a lovely blend for your home or office.

STORAGE Keep in a convenient location if you plan to use it up within a few weeks; otherwise, keep in a cool, dark place for up to a year.

## Grapefruit-Ylang-Ylang Diffusion

Makes 36 treatments

Fresh, tangy grapefruit combines with grounding chamomile and sweet ylang-ylang to delight your senses and decrease your stress level. This blend is an excellent one for wearing in an aromatherapy pendant.

48 drops grapefruit essential oil
32 drops Roman chamomile essential oil
28 drops ylang-ylang essential oil

1. In a small bottle, combine all the ingredients. Shake well to blend. With the cap secured, allow the different scents to marry for at least 24 hours before use.

2. Add 3 drops of the blend to your diffuser according to the manufacturer's instructions. Run the diffuser nearby. Repeat as needed.

# SUNBURN

While prevention is the best medicine, sunburns can and do happen. Aromatherapy treatments help by easing the pain and promoting faster healing. When applied immediately, they sometimes prevent the skin from peeling.

## Lavender-Cucumber Seed Spray

*Makes about 8 ounces*

Alongside aloe vera, soothing lavender and cucumber seed essential oils help take the sting out of sunburned skin while promoting faster healing. Meanwhile, witch hazel offers a welcome cooling sensation.

3 ounces distilled water
3 ounces witch hazel
2 ounces aloe vera gel
40 drops lavender essential oil
20 drops cucumber seed essential oil

1. In a bottle with a fine-mist spray top, combine all the ingredients. Shake well to blend, and then shake again before each use.

2. Apply 1 spritz to each burned area, using more as needed and ensuring that you cover the entire sunburn. Repeat hourly as needed.

STORAGE If you like, you can keep this spray in the refrigerator for an intense cooling sensation upon application; otherwise, keep in a cool, dark place.

## Helichrysum Milk Bath

Makes 4 treatments

Helichrysum essential oil combines with comforting, protein-rich powdered goat milk to soothe burning and help compromised skin heal.

**2 cups powdered goat milk**
**20 drops helichrysum essential oil**

3. In a large bowl, combine the ingredients. Whisk to blend thoroughly.

4. Sift the powder into another bowl to break up any lumps, and then transfer the blend to a jar.

5. Draw a lukewarm bath and add ½ cup of the blend to the tub, using your hand to stir it in. Soak in the bath for 15 to 20 minutes. Repeat once daily to encourage your skin to heal.

## Geranium-Lavender Sunburn Gel

Makes about 4 ounces

Geranium and lavender combine with cool aloe vera gel to ease sunburn pain and help skin heal a bit faster. If you can get this gel onto your skin as soon as you notice a burn forming, you may be able to prevent peeling.

**3 ounces aloe vera gel**
**2 tablespoons fractionated coconut oil**
**20 drops lavender essential oil**
**12 drops geranium essential oil**

1. In a large bowl, combine all the ingredients. Whisk to blend thoroughly, and then transfer the gel to a jar.

2. Apply 1 teaspoon of the blend to the affected area, using a little more or less as needed. Repeat two to three times daily until the skin is healed.

STORAGE If you like, you can keep this gel in the refrigerator for an intense cooling sensation upon application; otherwise, keep in a cool, dark place.

# SWOLLEN FEET

Swollen feet can happen after a long day of walking or extensive periods spent working at your desk. Aromatherapy treatments provide relief by targeting inflammation and encouraging overworked tissues to relax.

## Refreshing Grapefruit Lotion

Makes about 8 ounces

Not only does grapefruit essential oil smell fantastic, but it also helps decrease swelling by encouraging tissues to release excess water. May Chang promotes healing while adding an interesting note to the blend.

**8 ounces unscented body lotion
or hand cream**
**40 drops grapefruit essential oil**
**10 drops May Chang essential oil**

1. In a large bowl, combine all the ingredients. Whisk to blend thoroughly, and then transfer the lotion to a jar or back to its original container.

2. Apply 1 teaspoon of the lotion to your feet and ankles. Use a little more or less as needed, and then take 30 minutes to relax while elevating your feet, if possible. Use as often as you like, especially after a foot soak.

STORAGE Keep this lotion in a convenient location if you plan to use it all within two weeks; otherwise, keep it in a glass bottle or jar in a cool, dark place.

## Lemon-Juniper Soak and Massage

Makes 1 treatment

Fresh-smelling lemon combines with fragrant juniper essential oil and refreshing ice water to bring swelling down. You can use cool water for this treatment if you'd rather not dip your feet in ice water.

2 gallons cold water
10 ice cubes
10 drops juniper essential oil
10 drops lemon essential oil

1. In a basin that's large enough to accommodate both of your feet, combine all the ingredients.

2. Seat yourself comfortably in front of the basin and soak your feet for 15 to 20 minutes.

3. Dry your feet thoroughly, and then rub your feet with Refreshing Grapefruit Lotion or Lavender-Tea Tree Balm.

4. Relax with your feet elevated for at least 30 minutes. Repeat as needed.

## Lavender-Tea Tree Balm

Makes about 4 ounces

Lavender and tea tree essential oils help compromised tissue heal while delivering soothing relief from stiff, sore feet. This treatment is a fantastic one to try after a cool footbath.

2 ounces shea butter
1 ounce coconut oil, melted
1 ounce beeswax, melted
60 drops lavender essential oil
20 drops tea tree essential oil
10 drops peppermint essential oil
10 drops vitamin E oil

1. In a large bowl, combine all the ingredients. Whisk to blend thoroughly.

2. Pour the balm into a jar and allow it to cool completely before capping.

3. With your fingertips, apply a dime-size amount to each foot. Massage your feet firmly, beginning with your toes and working your way toward the ankles. Elevate your feet for 30 minutes if you have time, and repeat as needed.

# TENDINITIS

Tendinitis occurs after repeated stress to a tendon, often as the result of sports or repetitive motions that take place during work or electronics use. Aromatherapy treatments provide pain relief while targeting inflammation; in the meantime, you can help yourself heal by giving the stressed tendon a break. See your doctor or physical therapist for additional treatment if pain persists.

## Benzoin-Lavandin Compress

Makes 1 treatment

Soothing lavandin and benzoin combine with an ice pack or heating pad to bring swelling down and provide deep relief from pain. Begin your treatment with an ice pack. After the first three days of recovery, you can alternate between hot and cold, if you'd like.

½ teaspoon coconut oil
3 drops lavandin essential oil
2 drops benzoin essential oil

1. In the palm of your hand, combine all the ingredients.
2. Apply the blend to the painful tendon, and massage the area.
3. Wrap an ice pack in a towel and apply it to the injured area. Leave the pack in place for 15 to 20 minutes, and repeat the treatment at least three times daily during the first 3 days of recovery.
4. Once the swelling has subsided, apply the blend to the affected area and cover with a warm heating pad, following the manufacturer's instructions for safe use. The heat and essential oils combine to encourage greater circulation, which speeds the healing process.

## Peppermint-Lime Gel

Makes about 4 ounces

Brisk peppermint and uplifting lime penetrate deep, soothing discomfort while promoting faster healing.

3½ ounces aloe vera gel
1 tablespoon fractionated coconut oil
20 drops lavender essential oil
12 drops lemon verbena essential oil

1. In a large bowl, combine all the ingredients. Whisk to blend thoroughly, and then transfer the gel to a jar.

2. Apply 1 teaspoon of the blend to the affected area, using a little more or less as needed. Repeat two to three times daily, either alone or with an ice pack or heating pad.

STORAGE If you like, you can keep this gel in the refrigerator for an intense cooling sensation upon application; otherwise, keep in a cool, dark place.

## Helichrysum-Spruce Balm

Makes about 2 ounces

Fresh, fragrant spruce combines with soothing helichrysum, delivering relief from intense discomfort while encouraging compromised tissue to heal faster. Use this blend with an ice pack or heating pad, or apply it at bedtime.

1 tablespoon coconut oil, melted
1 tablespoon hemp oil
1 tablespoon shea butter
1 tablespoon sweet almond oil
12 drops helichrysum essential oil
24 drops spruce essential oil

1. In a medium bowl, combine all the ingredients. Whisk to blend thoroughly, and then transfer the balm to a small jar.

2. Apply 1 teaspoon of balm to the affected area, using a little more or less as needed. Massage gently until the blend has been absorbed. Repeat two to three times daily until pain subsides.

# TOENAIL FUNGUS

Toenail fungus causes discolored, thickened toenails, and is notoriously difficult to eradicate. Instead of reaching for potentially toxic drugstore remedies, give aromatherapy a chance to kill the fungus naturally.

## Tea Tree Neat Treatment

Makes 1 treatment

Tee tree essential oil is one of the most potent antifungal essential oils available, and it kills toenail fungus so well that many over-the-counter remedies rely on it. Be sure to conduct a patch test before using this neat treatment.

**1 drop tea tree essential oil**

1. Wash and dry the affected foot, and then use sterilized nail clippers to trim the infected nail straight across, removing as much of the fungus as possible without damaging the nail bed.

2. With a cotton swab, apply the tea tree essential oil to the top and sides of the toenail. Repeat two to three times daily until new, healthy nail replaces the old discolored nail.

## Lavender-Palmarosa Footbath

Makes 1 treatment

When added to a footbath, lavender and palmarosa essential oils kill fungus while softening and deodorizing.

1 gallon hot water
2 tablespoons Epsom salt
10 drops lavender essential oil
10 drops palmarosa essential oil

1. Use a pair of sterilized nail scissors to trim the affected toenails straight across, removing as much of the fungus as you can without damaging the nail bed.

2. In a shallow basin that's large enough to accommodate your foot, combine the hot water with the Epsom salt.

3. Add the essential oils to the basin, and then put the affected foot into the water. Allow it to soak for 10 to 15 minutes.

4. Dry your foot, and then apply a drop of lavender essential oil to each affected toenail. Repeat once daily until fungus is gone.

## Lemongrass Balm

Makes 1 ounce

Lemongrass essential oil is a potent antifungal agent, and its clean, uplifting aroma makes it a pleasure to use.

1 ounce fractionated coconut oil
6 drops lemongrass essential oil

1. In a small bottle or jar, combine the ingredients. Shake well to blend.

2. Use a pair of sterilized nail scissors to trim the affected toenails straight across, removing as much of the fungus as you can without damaging the nail bed.

3. With a cotton swab, apply 2 to 3 drops of the blend to each nail. Repeat two to three times daily until the fungus is gone.

# TOOTHACHE

Best practice is to get to the dentist as soon as possible when suffering from a toothache, but it can take time to get an appointment. While you're waiting, aromatherapy treatments can provide you with much-needed relief.

## Clove Bud Neat Treatment

Makes 1 treatment

Clove bud essential oil is such an effective numbing agent that it has a time-honored place in the history of dentistry. Just a drop delivers immediate relief. There's no need to worry about putting this in your mouth; your oral tissues will absorb it.

**1 drop clove bud essential oil**

1. With a pipette or medicine dropper, apply the essential oil directly to the painful tooth.

2. Breathe through your mouth to prevent saliva from washing the treatment away while it absorbs. You should be able to return to normal nose breathing within a minute or two. Repeat two to three times daily as needed.

## Synergistic Toothache Blend

Makes about 1 ounce

If tooth pain occurs because a wisdom tooth is erupting or you want to try something other than pain medication following an uncomfortable dental procedure, a topical application of clove bud, chamomile, and lemon can often bring comfort.

2 tablespoons sweet almond oil
90 drops German chamomile essential oil
30 drops clove bud essential oil
30 drops lemon essential oil

1. In a small bottle or jar, combine all the ingredients. Shake well to blend.

2. With your fingertips, apply ½ teaspoon of the blend to the outside portion of your cheek and/or jawline where pain is greatest. Massage well until the blend is absorbed.

## Chamomile-Peppermint Compress

Makes 1 treatment

Soothing chamomile and peppermint combine to ease dental pain quickly. A cotton ball holds the treatment in place. There's no need to rinse after this treatment; the small amount of oil in your mouth gets absorbed by the oral tissues.

6 drops distilled water
1 drop peppermint essential oil
1 drop Roman chamomile essential oil

1. In a small dish, combine all the ingredients. Saturate a cotton ball in the blend.

2. Apply the cotton ball to the affected tooth and keep it in place for 10 to 15 minutes. Repeat as needed to keep pain to a minimum.

# URINARY TRACT INFECTION (UTI)

Painful stinging upon urination and a constant feeling that you need to urinate even when your bladder is empty are two symptoms of UTIs. Aromatherapy treatments can help if you start to use them at the first sign of a UTI. If you have a fever or if the pain is getting worse, see your doctor.

## Lavender Rinse

Makes about 4 ounces

Lavender stops pain and kills bacteria, especially when applied in a strong concentration like this one. If you notice any irritation, stop using this treatment.

**4 ounces distilled water**
**40 drops lavender essential oil**

1. In a bottle or jar, combine the ingredients. Shake well to blend, and then shake again before each use.

2. After urinating, draw at least 10 milliliters of the blend into a dental syringe, and then gently rinse the urethral opening. Be careful not to let the syringe come into contact with your body. Repeat each time you urinate.

SUBSTITUTION TIP If you don't have a dental syringe, you can use a cotton ball or cosmetic pad to apply the remedy. Be sure to completely saturate the urethral opening.

## Synergistic Antiseptic Bath Salts

Makes 4 treatments

Bergamot, clove bud, juniper berry, eucalyptus, and cajuput are strong antiseptics that can help you fight off a UTI. The Epsom salt helps by encouraging your body to release toxins.

2 tablespoons fractionated coconut oil
16 drops bergamot essential oil
16 drops clove bud essential oil
16 drops juniper berry essential oil
12 drops cajuput essential oil
12 drops *Eucalyptus globulus* essential oil
4 cups Epsom salt

1. In a large bowl, combine the fractionated coconut oil and the essential oils. Add the Epsom salt and stir well to blend. Transfer the bath salts to a jar.

2. Fill your bathtub with 4 inches of hot water and dissolve 1 cup of bath salts in it. Soak in the bath for at least 20 minutes. Repeat once daily.

## Synergistic Antibacterial Massage Blend

Makes about 1 ounce

Fennel seed, tea tree, bergamot, cypress, and juniper berry essential oils offer strong antibacterial properties. Massaging your lower back and abdomen delivers the blend to the bladder.

1 ounce fractionated coconut oil
12 drops juniper berry essential oil
9 drops bergamot essential oil
9 drops tea tree essential oil
8 drops cypress essential oil
3 drops fennel seed essential oil

1. In a small bottle or jar, combine all the ingredients. Shake well to blend.

2. At the first sign of discomfort, apply 1 teaspoon of the blend to your lower abdomen and lower back, and massage the blend in well.

3. If you have time, cover your lower abdomen with a hot heating pad, following the manufacturer's instructions for safe use. Leave the heating pad in place for 15 minutes. Repeat twice daily.

# VAGINAL DRYNESS

The itching, irritation, and painful intercourse that accompany vaginal dryness are caused by a reduction in estrogen. Aromatherapy helps by reducing inflammation and irritation, and by lubricating sensitive vaginal tissue naturally.

## Healing Lavender-Helichrysum Oil

Makes 2 ounces

Lavender, helichrysum, and Roman chamomile essential oils combine with calendula herbal oil and wild yam herbal oil, moisturizing tissue and supporting healthy hormone levels.

1 ounce calendula herbal oil
1 ounce wild yam herbal liquid extract
7 drops lavender essential oil
5 drops Roman chamomile essential oil
4 drops helichrysum essential oil

1. In a bottle or jar, combine all the ingredients. Shake well to blend.
2. After bathing or showering, use your fingertips to apply ½ teaspoon of the blend to the vaginal area. Repeat once daily.

## Synergistic Vaginal Salve

Makes about 4 ounces

In this salve, frankincense, Roman chamomile, neroli, and sandalwood come together to heal compromised tissue, soothe inflammation, and support tissue regeneration.

3 ounces calendula herbal oil
1 tablespoon beeswax, melted
1 tablespoon fractionated coconut oil
10 drops frankincense essential oil
10 drops neroli essential oil
10 drops sandalwood essential oil
5 drops Roman chamomile essential oil

1. In a medium bowl, combine all the ingredients. Whisk to blend thoroughly, and then transfer the salve to a small jar.

2. After bathing or showering, use your fingertips to apply ½ teaspoon of the salve to the vaginal area. Repeat as needed for soothing moisture.

## Lubricating Chamomile-Rose Gel

Makes about 4 ounces

Rose, Roman chamomile, and sandalwood combine to stop itching and ease inflammation. Aloe vera gel provides relief from dryness while helping delicate tissue heal.

3½ ounces aloe vera gel
1 tablespoon fractionated coconut oil
14 drops sandalwood essential oil
7 drops Roman chamomile essential oil
5 drops rose otto or rose absolute

1. In a large bowl, combine all the ingredients. Whisk to blend thoroughly, and then transfer the gel to a jar.

2. Apply 1 teaspoon of the gel to the vaginal area, using a little more or less as needed. Repeat once daily or as needed.

# WARTS

A wart is a small skin growth with either a smooth or textured surface. Warts, which are caused by the human papillomavirus (HPV), are relatively common. The virus is highly contagious, so it's a good idea to treat a wart as soon as you notice one developing.

## Tea Tree Neat Treatment

Makes 1 treatment

Tea tree essential oil dries warts and kills the virus, encouraging skin to heal. Additionally, it serves as an antiseptic, preventing the area from becoming infected. Be sure to conduct a patch test before using this neat treatment.

**1 drop tea tree essential oil**

With a cotton swab, apply the tea tree essential oil directly onto the wart. Repeat two to three times daily until the wart disappears, usually within 1 to 2 weeks.

## Oregano Neat Treatment

Makes 1 treatment

Oregano kills the virus and irritates the wart tissue, causing it to shrink and fall off. Be very careful not to get any undiluted oregano essential oil onto the surrounding healthy skin. Be sure to conduct a patch test before using this neat treatment.

**2 drops carrier oil**
**1 drop oregano essential oil**

1. Coat the skin surrounding the wart with the carrier oil.

2. With a cotton swab, apply the oregano essential oil to the wart. Cover the wart with a bandage. Repeat the treatment one to two times daily until the wart falls off, usually within 5 to 10 days.

## Lavender Neat Treatment for Post-Wart Removal

Makes 1 treatment

When warts fall off, they often leave a small hole behind. Lavender provides protection from infection and encourages skin to heal faster. Be sure to conduct a patch test before using this neat treatment.

**1 drop lavender essential oil**

With a cotton swab, apply the lavender essential oil to the hole. Repeat the treatment two to three times daily until the site is healed.

# WATER RETENTION

Also known as *edema*, water retention occurs when fluid builds up in the body's tissues. The swelling and puffiness isn't just unsightly; it's also uncomfortable. Aromatherapy can help your body eliminate excess water, but if you suffer from this condition frequently, see your doctor to rule out a more serious underlying condition.

## Synergistic Diuretic Massage Gel

Makes about 4 ounces

A blend of grapefruit, geranium, and carrot seed essential oil acts as a natural diuretic, encouraging the body to shed excess water weight. Be sure to drink plenty of water; drinking water reassures your body that it's properly hydrated and encourages it to let go of the excess.

**3½ ounces aloe vera gel**
**1 tablespoon fractionated coconut oil**
**12 drops grapefruit essential oil**
**8 drops geranium essential oil**
**4 drops carrot seed essential oil**

1. In a large bowl, combine all the ingredients. Whisk to blend thoroughly, and then transfer the gel to a jar.

2. Apply 1 teaspoon of the gel to the area where swelling is most prevalent, working your way toward the heart. Repeat two to three times daily or as needed.

STORAGE If you like, you can keep this gel in the refrigerator for an intense cooling sensation upon application; otherwise, keep in a cool, dark place.

## Geranium-Juniper Berry Lotion

Makes about 8 ounces

Fragrant geranium, sweet orange, and juniper berry offer potent diuretic properties, plus they eliminate toxins and stimulate the body's lymphatic system. Use this lotion to encourage balance and prevent water retention.

8 ounces unscented body lotion
   or hand cream
20 drops geranium essential oil
10 drops juniper berry essential oil
10 drops sweet orange essential oil

1. In a large bowl, combine all the ingredients. Whisk to blend thoroughly, and then transfer the lotion to a jar or back to its original container.

2. Apply 1 teaspoon of the lotion to your hands, arms, and shoulders, and apply another ½ teaspoon to feet. Use a little more or less as needed, and feel free to apply the lotion to other body parts. Use as often as you like throughout the day, especially after washing your hands.

STORAGE Keep this lotion in a convenient location if you plan to use it all within two weeks; otherwise, keep it in a glass bottle or jar in a cool, dark place.

## Rosemary-Lemon Bath Salts

Makes 8 treatments

Delicious-smelling lemon, lavender, and rosemary essential oils combine with Epsom salt to encourage the body to release toxins.

2 tablespoons fractionated coconut oil
24 drops lemon essential oil
8 drops lavender essential oil
8 drops rosemary essential oil
4 cups Epsom salt

1. In a large bowl, combine the fractionated coconut oil and the essential oils. Add the Epsom salt and stir well to blend. Transfer the bath salts to a jar.

2. Draw a hot bath and add ½ cup of bath salts. Soak in the bath for at least 15 minutes. Repeat once daily or as needed.

# YEAST INFECTION

Unbearable itching, irritation, and yeasty-smelling discharge are among the signs of a yeast infection caused by *Candida albicans*. This fungus naturally inhabits the body, only causing problems when its population grows out of control.

## Lemon Salve

Makes about 1 ounce

Lemon essential oil is an effective antifungal agent that makes short work of a yeast infection. Blended with fractionated coconut oil, it also soothes the burning and itching.

**1 ounce fractionated coconut oil**
**16 drops lemon essential oil**

1. In a small bottle or jar, combine the ingredients. Shake well to blend.

2. Apply ½ teaspoon of salve to an applicator-free tampon and insert it into the vagina. Leave the tampon in place for 2 hours. Repeat three times daily until the yeast infection is gone.

## Synergistic Antifungal Douche

Makes 1 treatment

Rosemary, lavender, tea tree, and geranium combine with warm water and refreshing vinegar to kill excess yeast and soothe irritated tissue.

3 cups distilled water, lukewarm
2 tablespoons white vinegar
3 drops lavender essential oil
2 drops tea tree essential oil
2 drops rosemary essential oil
1 drop geranium essential oil

1. In a douche bag, combine all the ingredients. Shake to blend.

2. In the shower, use the douche, following the manufacturer's instructions. Repeat once daily until the yeast infection clears.

## Lavender-Tea Tree Tampon

Makes 1 treatment

Lavender and tea tree offer potent antifungal action, quickly ridding the vagina of excess yeast.

1 tablespoon distilled water, warm
2 drops lavender essential oil
2 drops tea tree essential oil

1. In a small bowl, combine all the ingredients. Soak an applicator-free tampon in the solution.

2. Insert the tampon into the vagina. Leave the tampon in place for 1 hour. Repeat twice daily until the yeast infection is gone.

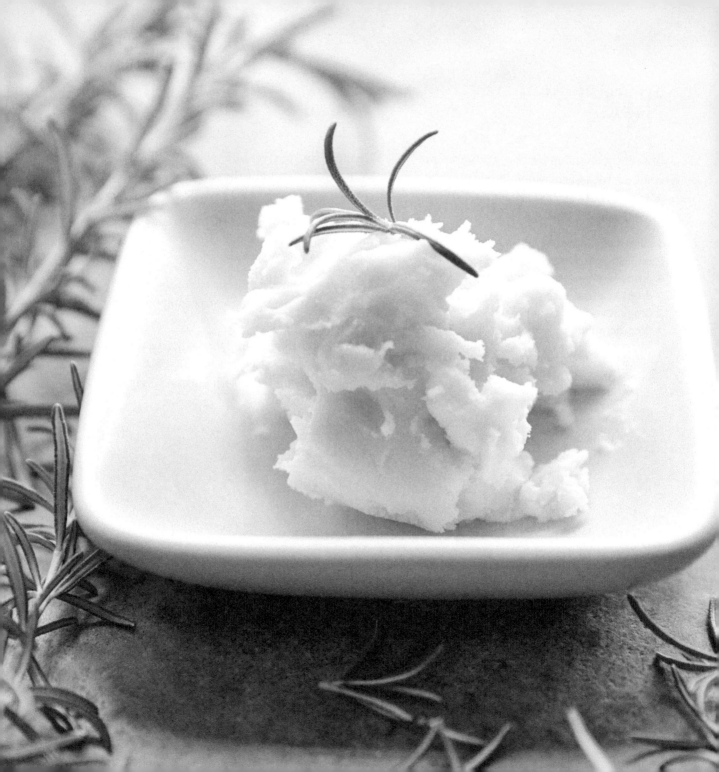

# FIVE

# Aromatherapy Recipes for Beauty

From frustrating pimples to painful cracked heels, common beauty problems are simple to solve with fragrant essential oils. In this chapter, you'll find 75 delightful aromatherapy treatments to help you look and feel your best, from head to toe. If you're looking for a way to deal with dandruff, heal chapped lips, banish split ends, or strengthen brittle nails, this is the place to find it.

As part of the planning process, remember to check each essential oil's profile to ensure that it is suitable for you. Essential oils should be capped tightly and stored in a cool, dark place. Unless otherwise noted, any treatments you make with essential oils that are not used immediately should be treated the same way.

# ACNE

Hormone fluctuations, clogged follicles, inflammation, bacteria, and a high-sugar/high-fat diet are some major contributors to acne. This condition shows up as inflamed skin, pimples, and clogged pores. Aromatherapy treatments work quickly and gently, leaving you with better-looking skin, naturally.

## Cooling Cucumber Seed-Tea Tree Toner

Makes about 4 ounces

Cucumber seed essential oil is a natural astringent, while tea tree essential oil kills bacteria. Witch hazel offers a cool, non-drying tingle.

**4 ounces alcohol-free witch hazel**
**20 drops cucumber seed essential oil**
**4 drops tea tree essential oil**

1. In a bottle or jar, combine all the ingredients, Shake well to blend, and then shake again before each use.

2. Apply ¼ teaspoon of the toner to a cotton cosmetic pad and gently swipe it all over your freshly washed face. Repeat morning and evening, before moisturizing.

## Lavender-Chamomile Steam

Makes 1 treatment

Lavender and chamomile essential oils work together to open your pores and detoxify your skin. This luxurious steam is ideal for use before exfoliation.

2 cups steaming hot water
3 drops lavender essential oil
3 drops Roman or German chamomile
essential oil

1. Pour the water into a large bowl, and then add the essential oils.

2. Sit comfortably in front of the bowl and drape a towel over your head and the bowl, creating a tent that concentrates the steam and vapors. Emerge to breathe cool air as needed. Try to spend 10 minutes exposing your face to the steam. Repeat once or twice weekly.

## Tea Tree Neat Treatment for Blemishes

Makes 1 treatment

Tea tree essential oil kills bacteria and shrinks blemishes quickly. Be sure to conduct a patch test before using this neat treatment.

1 drop tea tree essential oil

With a cotton swab, apply the essential oil to the blemish. Repeat the treatment on any additional blemishes. Repeat once or twice daily until blemishes are gone.

# AGE SPOTS

Flat brown, gray, or black patches of skin caused by exposure to the sun, age spots vary in size and are common in adults over age 40. While age spots are harmless, they can look similar to skin cancer; to be on the safe side, have them checked out by your doctor before proceeding with aromatherapy treatments.

## Synergistic Age Spot Salve

Makes about 1 ounce

Lavender, rose geranium, frankincense, and myrrh encourage the growth of healthy skin while helping fade age spots. Fractionated coconut oil helps prevent irritation by providing moisture.

1 ounce fractionated coconut oil
10 drops frankincense essential oil
10 drops lavender essential oil
10 drops myrrh essential oil
10 drops rose geranium essential oil

1. In a small bottle or jar, combine all the ingredients. Shake well to blend.

2. With a cotton swab, apply 1 drop of the salve to each age spot. Repeat two to three times daily until age spots fade.

## Lemon Mask

Makes 1 treatment

Lemon essential oil and yogurt encourage discolored skin to slough off quickly. Although this treatment is time-consuming, it is refreshing.

1 tablespoon plain yogurt
1 tablespoon oat flour
4 drops lemon essential oil

1. In a small bowl, combine all the ingredients. Whisk to blend thoroughly.

2. Wash and dry your face, and then apply the mask to your facial skin, being careful to avoid your eyes, as well as to any other areas where age spots are a concern. Leave the mask in place for 30 minutes, and relax.

3. Rinse the mask off with cold water, and then apply your favorite moisturizer. Repeat three times weekly until age spots fade.

## Sandalwood Neat Treatment

Makes 1 treatment

Sandalwood essential oil reduces the size and color of age spots, leaving fresh skin behind. Like other natural treatments, it takes several weeks to work. Be sure to conduct a patch test before using this neat treatment.

1 drop sandalwood essential oil

With a cotton swab, apply the sandalwood essential oil directly to the age spots. Add another drop if you need to cover a larger area. Repeat once or twice daily until age spots are gone.

# BRITTLE NAILS

Weakness, chipping, and splitting layers are some signs that you have brittle nails. You don't have to live with the problem; just like the rest of your skin, nails respond very well to aromatherapy.

### Frankincense Nail Balm

Makes about 1 ounce

Frankincense promotes strong, healthy skin and nail tissue, while rich jojoba oil provides much-needed moisture.

**1 ounce jojoba oil**
**50 drops frankincense essential oil**

1. In a small bottle or jar, combine the ingredients. Shake well to blend.

2. With a cotton swab, apply 1 drop of balm to each of your nails. Gently massage the blend into your nails, cuticles, and the surrounding tissue. Repeat three times weekly.

## Synergistic Nail-Strengthening Blend

Makes about 1 ounce

Lemon, peppermint, frankincense, and myrrh essential oils combine with nourishing vitamin E and wheatgrass oils to moisturize and strengthen nails.

1½ tablespoons wheat germ oil
½ tablespoon vitamin E oil
30 drops frankincense essential oil
20 drops lemon essential oil
20 drops myrrh essential oil
5 drops peppermint essential oil

1. In a small bottle or jar, combine all the ingredients. Shake well to blend.

2. With a cotton swab, apply 1 drop of the blend to each of your nails. Gently massage it into your nails, cuticles, and the surrounding tissue. Repeat once daily, preferably at bedtime.

## Lemon-Elemi Nail Soak

Makes 1 treatment

Brisk lemon and elemi essential oils kill any fungus that might be contributing to the problem, while warm water softens nails and prepares them to absorb the Frankincense Nail Balm (page 242) or the Synergistic Nail-Strengthening Blend (page 243).

1 cup warm water
1 drop elemi essential oil
1 drop lemon essential oil

1. In a medium bowl, combine the water and the essential oils.

2. Immerse your fingertips in the solution and soak your nails and cuticles for 5 minutes.

3. Pat your hands dry and immediately apply a moisturizing treatment. Repeat as often as you like.

# CALLUSES

Hard, thick skin on your feet, hands, or fingers is caused by things like hard handiwork, walking barefoot on rough surfaces, and even poorly fitting shoes. While painless, calluses are unsightly. Aromatherapy solves the problem by promoting softer skin.

## Lavender-Myrrh Massage

Makes about 2 ounces

Fragrant benzoin, myrrh, and lavender essential oils combine with sweet almond oil to deliver lasting softness.

2 ounces sweet almond oil
8 drops lavender essential oil
4 drops myrrh essential oil
2 drops benzoin essential oil

1. In a bottle or jar, combine all the ingredients. Shake well to blend.

2. With your fingertips, apply 3 drops of the blend to each callus. Gently massage it into the affected area and the surrounding tissue. Repeat once daily, preferably at bedtime.

## Synergistic Callus Blend

Makes about 2 ounces

This combination of rich carrot seed, palmarosa, myrrh, and benzoin essential oils, along with jojoba and vitamin E, softens thickened skin.

1½ ounces jojoba oil
1 tablespoon vitamin E oil
10 drops carrot seed essential oil
10 drops patchouli essential oil
5 drops benzoin essential oil
5 drops lavender essential oil
5 drops myrrh essential oil
5 drops Roman chamomile essential oil
4 drops bergamot essential oil
4 drops palmarosa essential oil

1.  In a bottle or jar, combine all the ingredients, Shake well to blend.

2.  With your fingertips, apply 3 drops of the blend to each callus. Gently massage it into the affected area and the surrounding tissue. Repeat two to three times daily, preferably applying the final treatment at bedtime.

## Rose Geranium Sugar Scrub

Makes about 4 ounces

Gritty brown sugar gently exfoliates the skin, while fractionated coconut oil and rose geranium smooth and heal it.

½ cup brown sugar
¼ cup fractionated coconut oil
20 drops rose geranium essential oil

1.  In a wide-mouth jar, combine all the ingredients. Stir well to combine.

2.  After bathing or showering, apply 1 teaspoon of the sugar scrub to the affected area and massage the skin, using firm circular strokes.

3.  Rinse with warm water, and then apply the moisturizer of your choice. Repeat three to four times weekly.

# CELLULITE

Cellulite is harmless, but its lumpy, bumpy appearance can make you feel self-conscious. Aromatherapy helps improve the appearance of cellulite, and a sensible diet, daily exercise, and adequate hydration create the right environment for lasting improvement.

## Synergistic Skin-Firming Lotion

Makes about 8 ounces

Lemon, cypress, rose geranium, and juniper essential oils encourage the body to release toxins while supporting lymphatic circulation and improving the appearance of cellulite.

7 ounces unscented body lotion
 or hand cream
1 ounce witch hazel
20 drops cypress essential oil
20 drops lemon essential oil
16 drops juniper essential oil
16 drops rose geranium essential oil

1. In a large bowl, combine all the ingredients. Whisk to blend thoroughly, and then transfer the lotion to a jar.

2. Apply 1 teaspoon of the lotion to areas where cellulite is a concern. Use a little more or less as needed, and feel free to apply the lotion to other body parts. Use as often as you like throughout each day, especially after bathing or showering.

STORAGE Keep this lotion in a convenient location if you plan to use it all within two weeks; otherwise, keep it in a glass bottle or jar in a cool, dark place.

## Synergistic Cellulite Massage Oil

Makes about 2 ounces

A combination of grapefruit, cypress, juniper berry, and lavender essential oils flush out toxins and encourage stretched skin to firm up. Apply this massage oil after exercising, when circulation is at its best.

2 ounces jojoba oil
30 drops cypress essential oil
30 drops grapefruit essential oil
30 drops juniper berry
10 drops lavender essential oil

1. In a bottle or jar, combine all the ingredients. Shake well to blend.
2. Apply 1 teaspoon of the massage oil to areas where cellulite is a concern, and massage the skin with firm, deep strokes. Repeat once daily.

## Anti-Cellulite Bath Salts

Makes 8 treatments

Cypress, fennel seed, juniper berry, and grapefruit essential oils combine with Epsom salt to encourage your body to release toxins and get rid of the excess water weight that makes cellulite look so puffy.

2 tablespoons fractionated coconut oil
16 drops fennel seed essential oil
16 drops juniper berry essential oil
8 drops cypress essential oil
8 drops grapefruit essential oil
4 cups Epsom salt

1. In a large bowl, combine the fractionated coconut oil with the essential oils. Add the Epsom salt and stir well to blend. Transfer the bath salts to a jar.
2. Draw a hot bath and add ½ cup of bath salts. Soak in the bath for at least 15 minutes. Repeat at least twice weekly.

# CHAPPED LIPS

Because your lips don't contain oil glands, they chap more easily than the rest of your skin does. Luxurious aromatherapy treatments help heal and moisturize your lips, and they don't contain any harmful petroleum products like many commercial lip balms do.

## Soothing Balsam of Peru Lip Gel

Makes 1 ounce

Balsam of Peru essential oil boosts circulation and helps compromised skin heal fast, while aloe and coconut oil deliver a much-needed touch of moisture.

5 teaspoons aloe vera gel
1 teaspoon fractionated coconut oil
6 drops balsam of Peru essential oil

1. In a small bowl, combine all the ingredients. Whisk to blend thoroughly, and then transfer the gel to a small jar.

2. With your fingertip, apply 2 drops of the gel to each lip. Allow the blend to absorb completely, and then apply a protective lip balm.

## Healing Frankincense Lip Balm

Makes 1 ounce

Frankincense soothes sore, chapped lips and helps them heal quickly, while a blend of rich oils provides protection from the elements.

½ tablespoon coconut oil, melted
½ tablespoon hemp oil
½ tablespoon shea butter
½ tablespoon sweet almond oil
12 drops frankincense essential oil

1. In a small bowl, combine all the ingredients. Whisk to blend thoroughly, and then transfer the balm to a small jar.

2. Apply 1 to 2 drops to lips several times each day to heal and prevent chapping.

## Lavender-Peppermint Lip Salve

Makes 100 treatments

Refreshing peppermint and healing lavender combine with fractionated coconut oil to soothe irritation while offering a deep, moisturizing effect.

1 tablespoon fractionated coconut oil
8 drops lavender essential oil
1 drop peppermint essential oil

1. In a small bottle, preferably with a roll-on applicator, combine all the ingredients. Shake well to blend.

2. With your fingertips or the roller, apply 2 to 3 drops to lips. Reapply as needed throughout the day, and again at bedtime.

STORAGE Keep in a convenient location if you plan to use it up within a few weeks; otherwise, keep in a cool, dark place for up to a year.

# CRACKED HEELS

Unsightly and often painful, cracked heels aren't just a cosmetic problem—they expose your feet to bacteria that could lead to infection. Delightful aromatherapy treatments help reveal soft skin and improve the overall health of your feet.

## Lemon-Lavender Foot Soak

Makes 1 treatment

Lavender and lemon essential oils smell marvelous together, but that's not all: they also eliminate bacteria and soften skin, especially when combined with soothing Epsom salt.

1 gallon warm water
⅓ cup Epsom salt
8 drops lavender essential oil
6 drops lemon essential oil

1. In a basin large enough to accommodate your feet, combine all the ingredients. Soak your feet for 15 minutes while relaxing.

2. Use a scrub brush or pumice stone to exfoliate your heels, but don't dig deep into the cracks; concentrate just on the tough outer layer of skin.

3. Pat your feet dry and apply a moisturizer. Repeat three to four times weekly until cracked heels resolve.

## Patchouli-Tea Tree Foot Balm

Makes about 2 ounces

Patchouli, tea tree, and lavender essential oils make quick work of fungus and bacteria, while rich emollients can help make your feet feel as soft as a petal.

1 tablespoon coconut oil, melted
1 tablespoon olive oil
1 tablespoon shea butter
1 tablespoon sweet almond oil
16 drops lavender essential oil
12 drops patchouli essential oil
6 drops tea tree essential oil

1. In a medium bowl, combine all the ingredients. Whisk to blend thoroughly, and then transfer the balm to a small jar.

2. Apply 1 teaspoon of balm to each foot, and massage into cracked heels. Repeat once or twice daily until cracked heels resolve.

## Synergistic Overnight Foot Cream

Makes about 8 ounces

This synergistic blend includes benzoin, myrrh, and geranium; it addresses bacteria and fungi while helping sore cracked heels feel better quickly. Consider wearing socks to bed to help keep the treatment on your feet overnight. In the morning, your feet will feel much softer and less painful.

8 ounces shea butter
20 drops geranium essential oil
10 drops benzoin essential oil
10 drops myrrh essential oil
8 drops lavender essential oil
4 drops tea tree essential oil

1. In a large bowl, combine all the ingredients. Whisk to blend thoroughly, and then transfer the cream to a jar.

2. Apply 1 teaspoon of the cream to each foot, concentrating on the heels, just before getting into bed. Put on a pair of socks and settle in for the night. Repeat nightly until cracked heels resolve.

# DANDRUFF

While many view dandruff as a cosmetic problem, it's also an itchy condition that can cause much discomfort. Because dandruff can worsen when you're sick or stressed, relaxing aromatherapy shampoos prove helpful on multiple fronts.

## Synergistic Dandruff Shampoo

Makes about 8 ounces

Rosemary, lavender, and tea tree combine with a touch of refreshing peppermint to soothe itching and kill bacteria that contribute to dandruff. You can use this shampoo every time you wash your hair.

8 ounces unscented shampoo
20 drops lavender essential oil
20 drops peppermint essential oil
10 drops tea tree essential oil
5 drops rosemary essential oil

1. In a large bowl, combine all the ingredients. Whisk to blend thoroughly, and then pour the shampoo into a plastic squeeze bottle.

2. Wet your hair and apply 1 teaspoon of the shampoo to your hair, using a little more or less as needed. Lather briskly, and then rinse. Follow up with Peppermint-Rosemary Conditioner (page 253).

STORAGE Keep this shampoo in the shower if you plan to use it all within two weeks; otherwise, keep it in a glass bottle or jar in a cool, dark place.

## Thyme Hot Oil Treatment

Makes 1 treatment

Thyme soothes itching and kills bacteria, plus it penetrates hardened scalp oils. The warm olive oil makes this treatment a pleasure.

1 ounce olive oil, warm
10 drops thyme essential oil

1. In a small bottle or bowl, combine the ingredients. Shake or stir well to blend.

2. Apply the entire treatment to your scalp, working it in. Wrap your head in a towel, and leave the towel on for 10 minutes.

3. Wash and condition your hair as usual, and then allow it to air-dry before styling it. Repeat three to four times weekly.

## Peppermint-Rosemary Conditioner

Makes about 8 ounces

Peppermint, rosemary, and lavender soothe itching and help stop dandruff, while promoting healthy, shiny hair.

8 ounces unscented conditioner
25 drops peppermint essential oil
20 drops lavender essential oil
10 drops rosemary essential oil

1. In a large bowl, combine all the ingredients. Whisk to blend thoroughly, and then pour the conditioner into a plastic squeeze bottle.

2. After shampooing, apply 1 teaspoon of the conditioner to your hair, using a little more or less as needed. Massage it gently into your scalp, wait 1 minute, and then rinse with cool water. Repeat every time you wash your hair.

STORAGE Keep this conditioner in the shower if you plan to use it all within two weeks; otherwise keep it in a glass bottle or jar in a cool, dark place.

# DRY HAIR

Dry, damaged hair often has a dull appearance, and it is much less manageable than healthy hair. Moisturizing aromatherapy treatments help restore shine and smoothness. If possible, stop using heated styling tools and allow your hair to dry naturally.

## Moisturizing Geranium-Myrrh Shampoo

Makes about 8 ounces

Myrrh and geranium smell marvelous together, and they help strengthen hair. A touch of fractionated coconut oil provides softness and shine. You can use this shampoo every time you wash your hair.

7½ ounces unscented shampoo
1 tablespoon fractionated coconut oil
20 drops myrrh essential oil
20 drops geranium essential oil

1. In a large bowl, combine all the ingredients. Whisk to blend thoroughly, and then pour the shampoo into a plastic squeeze bottle.

2. Wet your hair and apply 1 teaspoon of shampoo to your hair, using a little more or less as needed. Lather briskly, and then rinse. Follow up with Clary Sage-Sandalwood Conditioner (page 255).

STORAGE Keep this shampoo in the shower if you plan to use it all within two weeks; otherwise, keep it in a glass bottle or jar in a cool, dark place.

## Clary Sage-Sandalwood Conditioner

Makes about 8 ounces

Clary sage stimulates the scalp, encouraging healthy new hair growth, while sandalwood softens hair and leaves an intoxicating fragrance behind.

8 ounces unscented conditioner
20 drops sandalwood essential oil
10 drops clary sage essential oil

1. In a large bowl, combine all the ingredients. Whisk to blend thoroughly, and then pour the conditioner into a plastic squeeze bottle.

2. After shampooing, apply 1 teaspoon of conditioner to your hair, using a little more or less as needed. Massage it gently into your scalp, wait 1 minute, and then rinse with cool water. Repeat every time you wash your hair.

STORAGE Keep this conditioner in the shower if you plan to use it all within two weeks; otherwise, keep it in a glass bottle or jar in a cool, dark place.

## Moisturizing Chamomile Hair Mask

Makes 1 treatment

Chamomile essential oil soothes your scalp while lending softness and shine to your hair.

1 ounce fractionated olive oil, warm
10 drops Roman chamomile essential oil

1. In a small bottle or bowl, combine the ingredients. Shake or stir well to blend.

2. Apply the entire treatment to your hair, working it in. Wrap your head in a towel, and leave the towel on for 10 minutes.

3. Wash and condition your hair as usual, and then allow it to air-dry before styling it. Repeat three to four times weekly as needed.

# DRY HANDS

Arid indoor air, cold weather, and frequent hand washing can add up to dry, cracked skin on your hands. Moisturizing aromatherapy treatments can make a big difference, especially when used daily.

## Skin-Softening Hand Soap

Makes about 8 ounces

Fragrant lavender, soothing coconut oil, and natural castile soap make a marvelous antibacterial blend that soothes dry skin while protecting you from germs.

⅓ cup unscented liquid castile soap
20 drops lavender essential oil
⅔ cup distilled water
1 teaspoon fractionated coconut oil

1. In a bottle or jar with a foaming pump, combine the castile soap and the essential oil. Add the distilled water and coconut oil, and stir with a thin utensil to blend.

2. Pump once for a dollop of foam, and wash your hands. Use as often as needed.

## Lavender-Rosewood Hand Cream

Makes about 4 ounces

Lavender and rosewood moisturize skin and repair cracked and chapped areas while providing you with a bit of protection from germs.

4 ounces unscented hand cream
10 drops lavender essential oil
10 drops rosewood essential oil

1. In a large bowl, combine all the ingredients. Whisk to blend thoroughly, and then transfer the cream to a jar.

2. Apply 1 teaspoon of the cream to your hands, using a little more or less as needed. Use as often as you like, especially after washing your hands.

## Soothing Hand Balm

Makes about 4 ounces

Lavender and helichrysum soothe and heal chapped, cracked hands, while rich emollients moisturize deeply. For an unusual, but effective, nighttime deep-moisturizing treatment, put a pair of socks over your hands after applying the balm and leave the socks on overnight.

1 ounce coconut oil, melted
1 ounce shea butter
1 ounce sweet almond oil
1 tablespoon fractionated coconut oil
32 drops lavender essential oil
24 drops helichrysum essential oil

1. In a medium bowl, combine all the ingredients. Whisk to blend thoroughly, and then transfer the balm to a jar.

2. Apply 1 teaspoon of the balm to your hands, and massage it in. Repeat as needed.

# DRY SKIN

Sun, wind, air conditioning, and cold tend to leave skin feeling dry and itchy. Stay away from very hot water while working to repair it, and enjoy these nourishing aromatherapy remedies.

## Moisturizing Chamomile Body Wash

Makes 8 ounces

Roman chamomile stimulates the skin's oil production, and it helps heal chapped and irritated areas.

5 ounces unscented liquid castile soap
2 ounces fractionated coconut oil
20 drops Roman chamomile essential oil

1. In a large bowl, combine all the ingredients. Whisk to blend thoroughly, and then pour the body wash into a plastic squeeze bottle.

2. Apply 1 teaspoon of body wash to a wet sponge or bath pouf, using a little more or less as needed. Lather briskly, and then rinse. Pat yourself dry and follow up with Soothing Benzoin-Myrrh Body Lotion (page 259).

STORAGE Keep this body wash in the shower if you plan to use it all within two weeks; otherwise, keep it in a glass bottle or jar in a cool, dark place.

## Soothing Benzoin-Myrrh Body Lotion

Makes about 8 ounces

Benzoin, myrrh, and elemi help repair compromised skin while promoting deep moisture. The lotion forms a barrier between dry air and delicate skin.

8 ounces unscented body lotion
20 drops myrrh essential oil
10 drops benzoin essential oil
10 drops elemi essential oil

1. In a large bowl, combine all the ingredients. Whisk to blend thoroughly, and then transfer the lotion to a jar or back to its original container.

2. Apply 1 teaspoon of the lotion to each area of dry skin, using a little more or less as needed. Use as often as you like to keep skin moisturized.

STORAGE Keep this lotion in a convenient location if you plan to use it all within two weeks; otherwise, keep it in a glass bottle or jar in a cool, dark place.

## Sweet Orange-Rose Geranium Body Oil

Makes about 8 ounces

Sweet orange and rose geranium nourish and protect dry skin while helping compromised tissue repair itself. Body oil seals in moisture after a bath or shower, helping you stay comfortable longer.

4 ounces jojoba oil
2 ounces sweet almond oil
2 ounces sesame oil
30 drops rose geranium essential oil
20 drops sweet orange essential oil
10 drops pre-diluted jasmine essential oil (optional)

1. In a medium bowl, combine all the ingredients. Whisk to blend thoroughly, and then pour the body oil into a plastic bottle with a pump top.

2. Shower or bathe as usual, but before drying off, stand on a towel and apply 1 teaspoon of body oil to your arms, legs, torso, hands, and feet, using a little more or less as needed.

3. Pat yourself dry, and then apply Soothing Benzoin-Myrrh Body Lotion (page 259). Repeat after every bath or shower for soft, silky skin.

STORAGE Keep this body oil near the shower if you plan to use it all within two weeks; otherwise, keep it in a glass bottle or jar in a cool, dark place.

# FOOT ODOR

Just about everyone experiences foot odor sometimes. A combination of sweat and bacteria is to blame for the vinegary, cheesy, or ammonia-like stink; luckily, aromatherapy treatments handle the problem quickly and leave your tootsies smelling fresh.

## Grapefruit-Spearmint Foot Spray

Makes about 8 ounces

Cheerful grapefruit and fresh spearmint combine with fungus-fighting tea tree to create a delightful fragrance for your feet.

7 ounces distilled water
1 ounce witch hazel
20 drops grapefruit essential oil
10 drops spearmint essential oil
5 drops tea tree essential oil

1. In a bottle with a fine-mist spray top, combine all the ingredients. Shake well to blend, and then shake again before each use.

2. Apply 1 spritz to each area you'd like to address. Repeat two to three times a day as needed.

## Peppermint-Eucalyptus Pedicure Lotion

Makes about 8 ounces

Peppermint and eucalyptus essential oils kill bacteria. Plus, they provide a fresh, uplifting scent while imparting a cool, pleasant tingle.

8 ounces unscented body lotion
  or hand cream
20 drops peppermint essential oil
10 drops lemon eucalyptus essential oil

1. In a large bowl, combine all the ingredients. Whisk to blend thoroughly, and then transfer the lotion to a jar or back to its original container.

2. Apply ½ teaspoon of the lotion to each foot. Use a little more or less as needed, and feel free to apply the lotion to your ankles and lower legs if you like. Use once or twice daily to keep feet smelling fantastic.

STORAGE Keep this lotion in a convenient location if you plan to use it all within two weeks; otherwise, keep it in a glass bottle or jar in a cool, dark place.

## Rosemary-Lavender Foot Powder

Makes 1 cup

Lavender and rosemary essential oils have antibacterial and antifungal properties, making them the natural choice for better-smelling feet.

2 ounces baking soda
40 drops lavender essential oil
10 drops rosemary essential oil
4 ounces non-GMO cornstarch
2 ounces rice flour
1 teaspoon of uncooked rice
  (optional, for humidity control)

1. In a large measuring cup, combine the baking soda and the essential oils. Whisk to blend thoroughly.

2. Sift the mixture into a medium bowl, and then add the cornstarch and rice flour. Whisk again. If you are in a humid climate, add the rice to keep the powder from clumping, and mix in well. Transfer the powder to a glass or metal sugar shaker.

3. Sprinkle about ½ teaspoon of the powder onto each foot. Be sure to get some powder between each of your toes, too. Repeat two to three times daily.

# INGROWN HAIR

An ingrown hair sometimes looks like a little dark spot on your skin, but when bacteria gets trapped below the surface, the skin around the hair swells and becomes inflamed. With a good scrub, it's easy to remove a hair that has grown back into the skin. Meanwhile, essential oils help prevent infection and calm inflammation.

## Peppermint Sugar Scrub

Makes about 4 ounces

Peppermint essential oil helps ease discomfort, while sugar and coconut oil work together to free trapped hair. When the hair emerges, you can pluck it out, shave it off, or leave it.

½ cup brown sugar
¼ cup fractionated coconut oil
20 drops peppermint essential oil

1. In a wide-mouth jar, combine all the ingredients. Stir well to blend.

2. After bathing or showering, apply 1 teaspoon of sugar scrub to the ingrown hair, and massage the area, using firm circular strokes.

3. Rinse with warm water. Repeat daily until the ingrown hair emerges.

## Lavender Neat Treatment

Makes 1 treatment

If an ingrown hair is inflamed, lavender essential oil helps stop the pain and kill bacteria. You can use this treatment alongside a sugar scrub, or apply it after using tweezers to remove the hair and washing the area. Be sure to conduct a patch test before using this neat treatment.

**1 drop lavender essential oil**

Apply the lavender essential oil by dripping it directly onto the ingrown hair from the bottle, being careful not to touch the bottle to the skin. Repeat once daily while irritation persists.

## Soothing Tea Tree Compress

Makes 1 treatment

Tea tree essential oil combines with soothing heat to ease pain and stop inflammation, while helping prevent infection.

**½ teaspoon fractionated coconut oil**
**2 drops tea tree essential oil**

1. In the palm of your hand, combine the ingredients.

2. Apply the blend to the site of the ingrown hair.

3. Relax and cover the area with a warm heating pad, following the manufacturer's instructions for safe use. Leave the heating pad in place for at least 15 minutes. Repeat two to three times daily while working to free an inflamed ingrown hair.

# KERATOSIS PILARIS

Also known as chicken skin, keratosis pilaris is typified by small, hardened bumps of built-up keratin that rises up from blocked hair follicles on the backs of your arms. In some cases, it affects the backs of the thighs and the buttocks, too. Exfoliating and moisturizing aromatherapy treatments work wonders, as long as you keep using them; unfortunately, they don't stop your body from producing more keratin than it needs.

## Lavender Sugar Scrub

Makes about 8 ounces

Lavender helps heal irritation, while sugar and coconut oil combine to exfoliate and moisturize your skin.

1 cup brown sugar
1 cup coconut oil, softened
10 drops lavender essential oil

1.  In a medium bowl, combine all the ingredients. Stir well to combine, and then transfer the scrub to a jar.

2.  Spend a few minutes in a warm, steamy shower, allowing your skin to soften and your pores to open up. Then apply 1 teaspoon of the sugar scrub to each affected area, using a little more or less as needed. Scrub the area, using firm, circular strokes.

3.  Rinse off with warm water and pat yourself dry. Follow up with your favorite moisturizer, and repeat three to four times weekly.

## Tangerine-Tagetes Balm

Makes about 4 ounces

Cheerful tangerine and crisp-smelling tagetes combine with rich emollients to nourish and moisturize the skin between exfoliation treatments.

2 ounces coconut oil, melted
1 ounce shea butter
1 ounce sweet almond oil
16 drops tangerine oil
12 drops tagetes essential oil

1. In a medium bowl, combine all the ingredients. Whisk to blend thoroughly, and then transfer the balm to a small jar.

2. Apply 1 teaspoon of the balm to each affected area, using a little more or less as needed. Massage gently until the mixture is completely absorbed. Repeat once daily, preferably at bedtime.

## Mandarin-Rose Geranium Lotion

Makes about 8 ounces

Zingy mandarin and sweet rose geranium soften and smooth your skin, while light lotion leaves no oily residue behind. This blend is ideal for daily use.

8 ounces unscented body lotion
20 drops mandarin essential oil
20 drops rose geranium essential oil

1. In a large bowl, combine all the ingredients. Whisk to blend thoroughly, and then transfer the lotion to a jar or back to its original container.

2. Apply 1 teaspoon of the blend to each affected area. Use a little more or less as needed, and feel free to apply the lotion to other body parts. Use as often as you like throughout each day to keep skin well hydrated.

SUBSTITUTION TIP If you plan to spend time in the sun, replace the mandarin essential oil with 10 drops of frankincense.

STORAGE Keep this lotion in a convenient location if you plan to use it all within two weeks; otherwise, keep it in a glass bottle or jar in a cool, dark place

# OILY HAIR

Not only does excess oil weigh down your hair, but it may also be accompanied by dandruff. Aromatherapy helps by balancing oil production and removing excess oil from your scalp, minus the chemicals found in many commercial hair products.

## Rosemary-Peppermint Shampoo

Makes about 8 ounces

Rosemary and peppermint make a fantastic-smelling combo; they also help eliminate excess oil from your scalp.

8 ounces unscented shampoo
20 drops peppermint essential oil
20 drops rosemary essential oil

1. In a large bowl, combine all the ingredients. Whisk to blend thoroughly, and then pour the shampoo into a plastic squeeze bottle.

2. Wet your hair and apply 1 teaspoon of the shampoo to your hair, using a little more or less as needed. Lather briskly, and then rinse. Follow up with Lavender-Tea Tree Conditioner (page 267).

STORAGE Keep this shampoo in the shower if you plan to use it all within two weeks; otherwise, keep it in a glass bottle or jar in a cool, dark place.

## Lavender-Tea Tree Conditioner

Makes about 8 ounces

Lavender and tea tree condition your hair but leave no oily residue behind. If dandruff is an issue for you, as is often the case when hair is oily, you'll be glad to know that this conditioner helps stop flaking as well.

8 ounces unscented oil-free conditioner
10 drops tea tree essential oil
20 drops lavender essential oil

1. In a large bowl, combine all the ingredients. Whisk to blend thoroughly, and then pour the conditioner into a plastic squeeze bottle.

2. After shampooing, apply 1 teaspoon of the conditioner to your hair, using a little more or less as needed. Massage it gently into your scalp, wait 1 minute, and then rinse with cool water.

STORAGE Keep this conditioner in the shower if you plan to use it within two weeks; otherwise, keep it in a glass bottle or jar in a cool, dark place.

## Dry Shampoo

Makes 8 ounces

Dry shampoo absorbs excess oil and leaves hair looking fresh. Peppermint essential oil provides a pleasant tingle and leaves a delightful fragrance behind.

**For light hair**
1 cup arrowroot powder
20 drops peppermint essential oil

**For dark hair**
½ cup arrowroot powder
½ cup cocoa powder
20 drops peppermint essential oil

1. In a large bowl, combine all the ingredients. Whisk to blend thoroughly. Sift the mixture into a second bowl to remove any lumps, and then transfer the powder to a jar.

2. Use a long-handled cosmetic brush to apply a very light dusting of powder to your scalp, focusing on just the areas where oiliness is a problem.

3. Use a fine-tooth comb or brush to work the powder away from your scalp. Repeat as needed.

PREFERENCE TIP Though the peppermint imparts a fresh smell, you can substitute the peppermint in this recipe with any preferred essential oil.

# OILY SKIN

Your skin produces oil to protect itself from outside elements, but the extra oil can feel heavy and uncomfortable while attracting impurities that can lead to acne. Aromatherapy helps bring your skin back into balance, leaving you feeling fresh and looking fantastic.

### Deep-Cleansing Lavender-Lemon Steam

Makes 1 treatment

Fragrant lavender and lemon essential oils work together to detoxify your skin without overdrying it. This luxurious steam is ideal for use before exfoliation.

**2 cups steaming hot water**
**3 drops lavender essential oil**
**3 drops lemon essential oil**

1. Pour the hot water into a large bowl, and then add the essential oils.

2. Sit comfortably in front of the bowl and drape a towel over your head and the bowl, creating a tent that concentrates the steam and vapors. Emerge to breathe cool air as needed. Try to spend 10 minutes exposing your face to the treatment. Repeat two to three times weekly.

## Cooling Spearmint-Strawberry Mask

Makes 1 treatment

Strawberries and spearmint gently exfoliate and tone your skin without causing irritation. This treatment takes a little bit of time, but the result is worth it.

2 ripe strawberries, mashed
1 drop spearmint essential oil

1. In a small bowl, combine the ingredients. Mash thoroughly with a fork to blend.

2. Spread the pulp on a facial mask sheet or a paper towel in which you've cut holes for your eyes and mouth.

3. Lie down comfortably and apply the mask to your face, pressing lightly to ensure that the pulp is in contact with your skin. Leave the mask in place for 15 minutes.

4. Rinse your face with water, pat dry, and then apply your favorite moisturizer. Repeat up to three times weekly.

SUBSTITUTION TIP If you dislike the idea of putting fruit on your face, you can blend the spearmint essential oil with 1 tablespoon of aloe vera gel instead.

## Refreshing Peppermint-Cucumber Seed Toner

Makes about 4 ounces

Crisp, cool peppermint combines with refreshing cucumber seed essential oil and witch hazel to create a toner that removes excess oil without causing irritation.

4 ounces alcohol-free witch hazel
12 drops cucumber seed essential oil
8 drops peppermint essential oil

1. In a bottle with a narrow neck, combine all the ingredients. Shake well to blend, and then shake again before each use.

2. Apply ¼ teaspoon of the toner to a cotton cosmetic pad and gently swipe it all over your freshly washed face. Repeat twice daily, following up with oil-free moisturizer, if you like.

# ORAL HYGIENE

While there's no denying the importance of regular visits to the dentist, it's also true that you don't need chemicals to keep your mouth clean and healthy. Give these refreshing recipes a try; they're like luxurious spa treatments for your teeth.

## Antibacterial Clove Bud Oil Pull

Makes 1 treatment

Oil pulling reduces plaque and bacteria, plus it helps strengthen your gums. Adding clove bud essential oil makes the treatment even more potent.

**1 teaspoon organic coconut oil**
**1 drop clove bud essential oil**

1. First thing in the morning, before eating or drinking anything, put the coconut oil in your mouth and allow it to melt.

2. With a dropper, drip the clove bud essential oil onto the coconut oil in your mouth.

3. Gently swish the oil around your mouth and between your teeth, as you would with a mouthwash, for 15 minutes. (You can perform other morning tasks while swishing.)

4. Spit the treatment into a paper towel and discard it. Repeat every morning.

SUBSTITUTION TIP If you dislike the taste of clove bud, you can try peppermint, spearmint, or lemon in its place.

## Herbal Dental Rinse

Makes 8 ounces

Uplifting peppermint, rosemary, and lavender boost your mood while killing harmful bacteria in your mouth and leaving you with fresh breath. Remember not to swallow the rinse.

7 ounces distilled water
1 ounce brandy
3 drops peppermint essential oil
1 drop lavender essential oil
1 drop rosemary essential oil

1. In a bottle or jar, combine all the ingredients. Shake well to blend, and then shake again before each use.

2. Swish with 1 teaspoon of the rise for 30 seconds to 1 minute, being careful not to swallow. Repeat two to three times daily, especially after meals and snacks.

PREFERENCE TIP If you would prefer an alcohol-free version of this rinse, simply omit the brandy and increase the water to 8 ounces.

## Antibacterial Dental Floss

Makes 1 treatment

Clove bud essential oil gives your dental floss a bacteria-killing boost while removing debris from between your teeth.

1 piece of unflavored dental floss
1 drop clove bud essential oil

1. Apply the clove bud essential oil to a cotton cosmetic pad, and pinch the pad over a piece of dental floss so that the essential oil comes into contact with it. Slowly pull the floss through the cosmetic pad.

2. Floss your teeth as usual. Repeat each time you floss.

# PUFFY EYES

Allergies, crying, overwork, or tiredness can lead to inflammation around the eyes. Puffiness goes away on its own after several hours, but you can use aromatherapy to help speed the process along.

## Helichrysum-Cucumber Seed Compress

Makes 1 treatment

Refreshing cucumber seed and helichrysum essential oils combine with ice cubes to shrink swollen tissue and provide a feeling of refreshment.

½ teaspoon distilled water
1 drop helichrysum essential oil
1 drop cucumber seed essential oil
2 ice cubes

1. In a small bowl, combine the water and the essential oils.

2. Soak 2 cotton cosmetic pads in the solution until saturated.

3. Lie down comfortably with your eyes closed, and gently place a pad over each eyelid. Top each pad with an ice cube. Leave the compress in place for 15 minutes. Repeat two to three times daily, if needed.

## Synergistic Eye Serum

Makes 100 treatments

Soothing cypress, frankincense, and Roman chamomile combine to calm the inflammation that causes puffy eyes.

1 tablespoon sweet almond oil
8 drops cypress essential oil
8 drops frankincense essential oil
2 drops Roman chamomile essential oil

1. In a small bottle, preferably with a roll-on applicator, combine all the ingredients. Shake well to blend.

2. With your fingertips or the roller, apply 1 drop of the serum to each swollen area below your eye. Gently massage the serum in, taking care not to get it in your eye or on sensitive eye tissue.

STORAGE Keep in a convenient location if you plan to use it up within a few weeks; otherwise, keep in a cool, dark place for up to a year.

## Lavender Eye Massage

Makes 1 treatment

Soothing lavender essential oil and nourishing rosehip oil combine to stop swelling and heal delicate tissue. If the puffy areas around your eyes have a purple or blue tone, this is a good remedy to try.

2 drops lavender essential oil
2 drops rosehip oil

1. In the palm of your nondominant hand, combine the ingredients.

2. With the ring finger of your dominant hand, gently dab a drop of the blend onto each swollen area. Using very light pressure, massage the area until the blend is fully absorbed. Repeat daily.

# RAZOR BUMPS

Shaving leaves you hair-free, but all too often, irritated red bumps are left behind. These simple aromatherapy treatments address the swelling, itchiness, and discomfort, leaving your skin looking smooth and healthy.

## Tea Tree Gel

Makes about 4 ounces

Antiseptic tea tree essential oil combines with soothing aloe vera gel to stop infection and ease inflammation quickly.

**4 ounces aloe vera gel**
**20 drops tea tree essential oil**

1. In a large bowl, combine the ingredients. Whisk to blend thoroughly, and then transfer the gel to a jar.

2. Apply 1 teaspoon of the blend to the affected area, using a little more or less as needed. Repeat two to three times daily whenever razor bumps are a problem.

STORAGE If you like, you can keep this gel in the refrigerator for an intense cooling sensation upon application; otherwise, keep in a cool, dark place.

## Honey-Lavender Mask

Makes 1 treatment

Honey and lavender offer antibacterial properties, plus they soothe the itching, reduce redness, and help bring swelling down.

**10 drops lavender essential oil**
**1 teaspoon honey**

1. With your fingertips or a cotton swab, apply the lavender essential oil directly to the affected area. Use additional drops if treating a large area or reduce the number of drops if treating a small area.

2. With your fingertips, apply the honey over the lavender essential oil. Use a little more or less as needed to cover the affected area. Leave the treatment in place for 10 to 15 minutes.

3. Rinse the area with cool water and pat dry. Repeat once or twice daily as needed.

## Lavender-Tea Tree Balm

Makes about 1 ounce

Soothing lavender and tea tree essential oils combine with antibacterial coconut oil to help prevent razor bumps on freshly shaved skin.

**1 ounce coconut oil, softened**
**24 drops tea tree essential oil**
**14 drops lavender essential oil**

1. In a medium bowl, combine all the ingredients. Whisk to blend thoroughly, and then transfer the balm to a jar.

2. After shaving, apply 1/2 teaspoon of the balm to the shaved area, and rub it in gently. Repeat each time you shave to prevent razor bumps.

# ROSACEA

Rosacea causes redness on the cheeks, chin, forehead, and nose, often with accompanying bumps and pimples. Avoiding triggers is the best way to prevent flare-ups, but when a flare-up occurs, aromatherapy can help bring your skin back to normal.

## Soothing Chamomile-Cypress Gel

Makes 4 ounces

German chamomile and cypress combine with peppermint to soothe inflammation, shrink swollen tissue, and promote cooling.

3½ ounces aloe vera gel
1 tablespoon fractionated coconut oil
6 drops cypress essential oil
6 drops German chamomile essential oil
4 drops peppermint essential oil

1. In a large bowl, combine all the ingredients. Whisk to blend thoroughly, and then transfer the gel to a jar.

2. Apply 1 teaspoon of the blend to the affected area, using a little more or less as needed. Repeat two to three times daily until the rosacea flare-up subsides.

STORAGE If you like, you can keep this gel in the refrigerator for an intense cooling sensation upon application; otherwise, keep in a cool, dark place.

## Cooling Cucumber-Geranium Toner

Makes 4 ounces

Both geranium and cucumber seed essential oils are natural astringents, and along with witch hazel, they help shrink swollen tissue and provide a pleasant tingle.

4 ounces alcohol-free witch hazel
8 drops cucumber seed essential oil
8 drops geranium or rose geranium
   essential oil

1. In a bottle or jar, combine all the ingredients. Shake well to blend, and then shake again before each use.

2. Apply ¼ teaspoon of the toner to a cotton cosmetic pad and gently swipe it all over your freshly washed face. Repeat morning and evening, before moisturizing.

## Synergistic Rosacea Blend

Makes 4 ounces

Sweet orange, fragrant geranium, and soothing helichrysum combine with grapefruit and cypress to shrink swelling and help irritated skin heal.

4 ounces calendula oil
4 drops helichrysum essential oil
3 drops cypress essential oil
2 drops geranium or rose geranium
   essential oil
2 drops grapefruit essential oil
2 drops lavender essential oil
2 drops sweet orange essential oil

1. In a bottle or jar, combine all the ingredients. Shake well to blend.

2. With a cotton cosmetic pad, apply ½ teaspoon of the blend to your freshly washed face, targeting all areas where rosacea is present. Use a little more or less as needed. Repeat twice daily.

# SPIDER VEINS/ VARICOSE VEINS

Varicose veins are twisted red, blue, and purple blood vessels that can be seen through skin; they are often uncomfortable and even painful. Spider veins are their smaller counterparts. In most cases, astringent aromatherapy treatments can reduce their appearance and provide relief from discomfort. Severe varicose veins usually require surgical intervention.

## Synergistic Body Cream for Varicose Veins

Makes about 8 ounces

Rich emollients combine with helichrysum, cypress, lemon, and fennel seed to reduce inflammation and swelling.

**4 ounces coconut oil, softened**
**4 ounces unscented body lotion**
**1 tablespoon vitamin E oil**
**15 drops cypress essential oil**
**15 drops helichrysum essential oil**
**15 drops lemon essential oil**
**12 drops fennel seed essential oil**

1. In a large bowl, combine all the ingredients. Whisk to blend thoroughly, and then transfer the cream to a jar.

2. Apply 1 teaspoon of the cream to the affected areas. Use a little more or less as needed, and feel free to apply the cream to other body parts. Use as often as you like throughout each day, especially after bathing and before bed.

## Cooling Juniper Berry Gel

Makes about 4 ounces

Bracing juniper, peppermint, and clary sage essential oils combine with soothing aloe vera gel to cool and comfort tired legs while helping shrink swollen vessels over time.

3½ ounces aloe vera gel
1 tablespoon fractionated coconut oil
20 drops clary sage essential oil
20 drops juniper berry essential oil
12 drops peppermint essential oil

1. In a large bowl, combine all the ingredients. Whisk to blend thoroughly, and then transfer the gel to a jar.

2. Apply 1 teaspoon of the gel to the affected area, using a little more or less as needed. Repeat two to three times daily to ease swelling and discomfort.

STORAGE If you like, you can keep this gel in the refrigerator for an intense cooling sensation upon application; otherwise, keep in a cool, dark place.

## Frankincense-Geranium Massage

Makes 1 treatment

Massaging spider or varicose veins with astringent essential oils can help reduce swelling, particularly if you make it part of your daily routine.

1 teaspoon jojoba oil
5 drops frankincense essential oil
5 drops geranium essential oil

1. In the palm of your hand, combine all the ingredients.

2. Apply the blend to the affected area, and gently massage it in, gradually working your way toward the heart. Repeat twice daily, elevating your feet for 15 minutes afterward.

# SPLIT ENDS

Heated styling tools and rough handling are two of the main causes of split ends. While the only real way to get rid of them is to get a trim, aromatherapy treatments can help improve your look by smoothing and softening hair to make it more manageable.

## Sandalwood Split-End Gel

Makes 1 ounce

Sandalwood softens and strengthens hair, which helps prevent breakage and keeps your split ends from getting worse. Just a little bit of this gel goes a long way.

1 ounce aloe vera gel
10 drops sandalwood essential oil

1. In a small bowl, combine the ingredients. Whisk to blend thoroughly, and then transfer the gel to a jar.
2. With your fingertips, apply 1 drop of gel to each area where split ends are present. Repeat the treatment two to three times daily as needed.

## Synergistic Split-End Conditioner

Makes 2 ounces

Rosemary, peppermint, geranium, lavender, and clary sage combine with rich coconut oil and sweet almond oil to nourish and soften hair between cuts.

3 tablespoons coconut oil, softened
1 tablespoon sweet almond oil
2 drops geranium essential oil
2 drops lavender essential oil
2 drops peppermint essential oil
1 drop clary sage essential oil
1 drop rosemary essential oil

1. In a small bowl, combine all the ingredients. Whisk to blend thoroughly, and then transfer the conditioner to a jar.

2. Before showering, apply the conditioner to the tips of your hair. Allow it to sit for 15 minutes, then wash and condition hair as usual.

## Ultra-Rich Conditioning Mask

Makes 1 treatment

A combination of helichrysum, myrrh, and lavender essential oils in a base of rich olive oil delivers intense moisture to hair and helps improve the appearance of split ends.

2 ounces olive oil
4 drops lavender essential oil
2 drops helichrysum essential oil
2 drops myrrh essential oil

1. In a medium bowl, combine all the ingredients. Whisk to blend thoroughly.

2. Before showering, apply the mask to your hair, completely saturating it. Allow it to sit for 15 minutes, then wash and condition hair as usual.

# STRETCH MARKS

When skin distends or contracts rapidly due to pregnancy, an adolescent growth spurt, or weight gain/loss, combined with hormonal changes that occur at the same time, the off-color striations we know as stretch marks develop. Aromatherapy treatments can't make them disappear overnight, but they can help bring your skin closer to its former smooth appearance.

## Galbanum Cream

Makes about 8 ounces

Cocoa butter and shea butter moisturize deeply, while galbanum strengthens skin and improves its appearance.

**4 ounces cocoa butter**
**4 ounces shea butter**
**32 drops galbanum essential oil**

1. In a large bowl, combine all the ingredients. Blend with an electric hand mixer, and then transfer the cream to a jar.

2. Apply 1 teaspoon of the cream to the affected areas, using a little more or less as needed. Repeat once or twice daily until stretch marks fade.

## Mandarin-Helichrysum Balm

Makes about 4 ounces

Delightful mandarin and soothing helichrysum nourish skin, while cocoa butter and avocado oil add moisture.

3 ounces cocoa butter
1 ounce avocado oil
12 drops mandarin essential oil
8 drops helichrysum essential oil

1. In a large bowl, combine all the ingredients. Blend with an electric hand mixer, and then transfer the balm to a jar.

2. Apply 1 teaspoon of the balm to the affected areas, using a little more or less as needed. Repeat once or twice daily until stretch marks fade.

## Geranium-Neroli Cream

Makes about 8 ounces

Neroli and geranium help damaged skin heal, and when applied to fresh, purple stretch marks, they can help minimize the appearance of the light-colored scars that appear later.

6 ounces shea butter
2 ounces jojoba oil
20 drops geranium or rose geranium essential oil
10 drops neroli essential oil

1. In a large bowl, combine all the ingredients. Blend with an electric hand mixer, and then transfer the cream to a jar.

2. Apply 1 teaspoon of the cream to the affected areas, using a little more or less as needed. Repeat once or twice daily until stretch marks fade.

# THINNING HAIR

Anyone can suffer from premature hair loss, with factors such as heredity, stress, and hormonal imbalances playing influential roles. Aromatherapy helps by stimulating the blood vessels that supply hair follicles, nourishing them and encouraging hair regrowth.

## Rosemary-Cucumber Seed Scalp Massage

Makes about 4 ounces

Rosemary and cucumber seed stimulate the blood vessels in the scalp and encourage stress relief, while fractionated coconut oil helps carry the treatment deep into the skin.

**4 ounces fractionated coconut oil**
**30 drops rosemary essential oil**
**20 drops cucumber seed essential oil**

1. In a plastic squeeze bottle, combine all the ingredients. Shake well to blend.

2. Apply 1 tablespoon of the blend to your scalp. With your fingertips, massage your scalp vigorously in tight circular motions.

3. Wash and condition your hair with Rosemary-Thyme Shampoo (page 285) and Atlas Cedarwood-Lavender Conditioner (page 285). Repeat once daily.

## Rosemary-Thyme Shampoo

Makes about 8 ounces

Rosemary and thyme essential oils stimulate the scalp and promote good circulation.

7½ ounces unscented shampoo
1 tablespoon fractionated coconut oil
20 drops rosemary essential oil
20 drops thyme essential oil

1. In a large bowl, combine all the ingredients. Whisk briskly to blend, and then pour the shampoo into a plastic squeeze bottle.

2. Wet your hair and apply 1 teaspoon of shampoo to your hair, using a little more or less as needed. Lather briskly, massaging with your fingertips, and then rinse. Follow up with Atlas Cedarwood-Lavender Conditioner.

STORAGE Keep this shampoo in the shower if you plan to use it all within two weeks; otherwise, keep it in a glass bottle or jar in a cool, dark place.

## Atlas Cedarwood-Lavender Conditioner

Makes about 8 ounces

Fragrant Atlas cedarwood and relaxing lavender promote good circulation and help you relax while promoting healthy, shiny hair.

8 ounces unscented conditioner
25 drops Atlas cedarwood essential oil
20 drops lavender essential oil

1. In a large bowl, combine all the ingredients. Whisk briskly to blend, and then pour the conditioner into a plastic squeeze bottle.

2. After shampooing, apply 1 teaspoon of the conditioner to your hair, using a little more or less as needed. Gently massage it into your scalp, wait 1 minute, and then rinse with cool water.

STORAGE Keep this conditioner in the shower if you plan to use it all within two weeks; otherwise, keep it in a glass bottle or jar in a cool, dark place.

# WRINKLES

Wrinkles are a byproduct of our facial expressions, repetitive facial movements, and sun damage. Most people will develop wrinkles at some point. Aromatherapy can help firm skin and reduce the appearance of wrinkles and crow's feet, especially if you make a point of taking preventive action.

## Synergistic Firming Serum

Makes about 2 ounces

Refreshing cucumber seed essential oil joins forces with others to tighten, moisturize, balance, and even out your skin's appearance. Rosehip oil is a must-have for this treatment, because it increases collagen production and encourages cell regeneration.

1 ounce sweet almond oil
1 ounce rosehip seed oil
10 drops cypress essential oil
10 drops geranium essential oil
7 drops frankincense essential oil
3 drops cucumber seed essential oil

1. In a bottle with an orifice reducer, combine all the ingredients. Shake well to blend.

2. With your fingertips, apply 2 to 3 drops of serum to your freshly washed face. Use a little more or less, so that the serum covers your entire face and absorbs completely. Treat your neck and décolletage areas, if you like. Repeat once or twice daily.

## Synergistic Smoothing Blend

Makes about 2 ounces

Rosehip oil delivers potent elemi, lavender, and neroli oils deep into skin, helping reduce the appearance of fine lines and wrinkles.

2 ounces rosehip oil
10 drops elemi essential oil
10 drops lavender essential oil
10 drops neroli essential oil

1. In a bottle with an orifice reducer, combine all the ingredients. Shake well to blend.

2. With your fingertips, apply 2 to 3 drops to your freshly washed face. Use a little more or less so that the blend covers your entire face and absorbs completely. Treat your neck and décolletage areas, if you like. Repeat once or twice daily.

## Rosewood-Patchouli Toner

Makes about 4 ounces

Rosewood and patchouli nourish your skin and promote healthy circulation, while rose water provides a skin-softening effect.

4 ounces rose water
10 drops rosewood essential oil
10 drops patchouli essential oil

1. In a bottle or jar, combine all the ingredients. Shake well to blend, and then shake again before each use.

2. Apply ¼ teaspoon of the toner to a cotton cosmetic pad and gently swipe it all over your freshly washed face. Repeat morning and evening, before moisturizing.

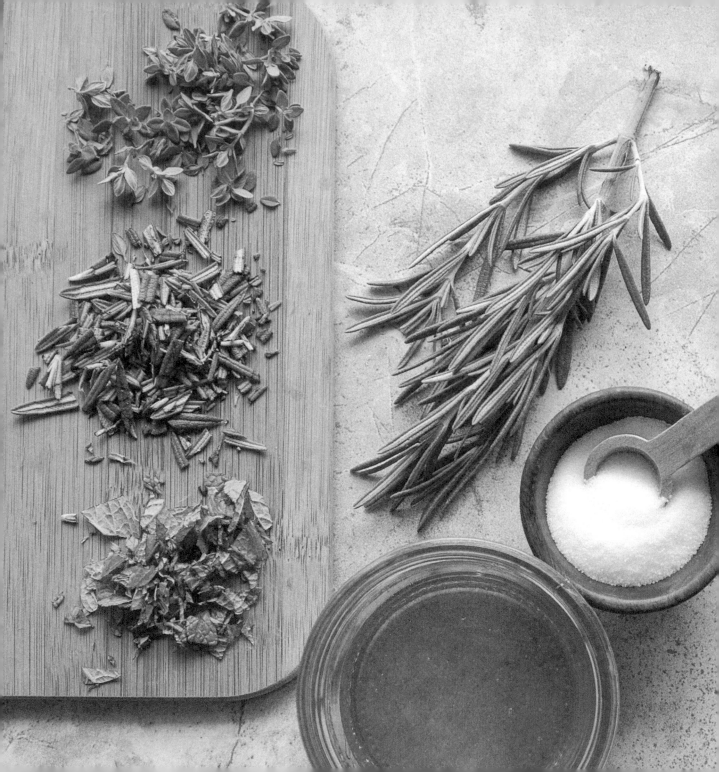

# SIX

# Aromatherapy Recipes for the Home

Aromatherapy isn't limited to treating ailments or enhancing your natural beauty. In this chapter, you'll discover ways to incorporate powerful essential oils into your everyday life. If you are interested in clearing your cupboards of toxins and making your home a healthier, more fragrant place to be, then this chapter was written with you in mind. Delightful air fresheners, simple ways to keep pests away, and family-friendly insect repellents are just a few of the things you'll discover here.

Essential oils should be capped tightly and stored in a cool, dark place. Unless otherwise noted, any products you make with essential oils that are not used immediately should be treated the same way.

# AIR FRESHENER

Commercial air fresheners may smell nice, but they often contain dangerous chemicals. Luckily, you can banish odors with aromatherapy instead and enjoy health benefits along the way. You can use these fun DIY air fresheners as inspiration for creating your own fragrant mists.

## Fresh Summer Breeze Spray

Makes about 4 ounces

Pure, fresh floral notes blend with a touch of citrus to give your home a fresh, sunny scent while promoting positive emotions.

4 ounces distilled water
40 drops geranium essential oil
40 drops mandarin essential oil
60 drops lavender essential oil
20 drops Roman chamomile essential oil

1. In a bottle with a fine-mist spray top, combine all the ingredients. Shake well to blend, and then shake again before each use.

2. Spritz the air a few times. Repeat as needed.

PREFERENCE TIP If you prefer a romantic floral scent rather than a citrusy one, omit the mandarin and add 10 drops of ylang-ylang to the blend.

## Spicy Autumn Room Deodorizer

Makes 1 air freshener

Bathrooms, baby-changing areas, and bedrooms are just a few places to put these simple, effective deodorizers. You can use them in your car, too.

10 drops clove bud essential oil
8 drops ginger essential oil
6 drops cinnamon leaf essential oil
5 drops sweet orange essential oil
2 drops lemon essential oil
1 drop anise essential oil
½ cup baking soda

1. In an 8-ounce canning jar, combine all the ingredients, using a fork to blend. Cover the jar opening with cheesecloth and secure with the ring, leaving the lid off.

2. Place the jar in the area where odor control is needed, positioning it out of reach of small children and pets. Stir the powder every 2 to 3 days to revive the scent, and add more essential oil to refresh the fragrance. Discard after refreshing two to three times.

SUBSTITUTION TIP If you're missing one or two of these essential oils, increase the number of drops of one of the other essential oils to compensate. You can also make your own signature scent by using 30 to 40 drops of any essential oil or blend in this recipe.

## Plug-In Air Freshener Refill

Makes 1 reusable refill

Plug-in air fresheners are convenient and smell nice, but most choices you'll find in your local store contain toxins. Instead of one of these, consider freshening your home with a plug-in that's made specifically for use with aromatherapy.

1 aromatherapy plug-in
5 to 7 drops of your favorite essential oil or blend

Apply the essential oil or blend to the diffuser's pad, and then plug in, following the manufacturer's instructions for safe use.

PREFERENCE TIP If this doesn't appeal to you or if you don't already have one of these devices, look for a plug-in that's made specifically for use with aromatherapy. Apply 5 to 7 drops of the essential oil or blend of your choice to the diffuser's pad and plug-in, following the manufacturer's instructions.

# ANT REPELLENT

No one likes to discover that ants have infested an area of their home and may be quick to reach for dangerous pesticides. Fortunately, aromatherapy offers a fragrant, nontoxic solution to ant problems.

## Ant-Eliminating Lavender Neat Treatment

Makes 1 treatment

Lavender essential oil is an ant irritant, so if ants find it along their route, they'll look elsewhere. This treatment works best when you first notice just a few ants. Use Peppermint-Tea Tree Ant Spray (page 293) or Peppermint Ant Killer (page 293) for more serious infestations.

**3 drops lavender essential oil (per entry point)**

1. Watch the ants as they make their way from one place to the next, but don't disturb them. If you follow their path, you'll find their entry point usually along a doorframe or within a windowsill.

2. Look outside in that area to see if you can find a corresponding trail of ants entering your home. If so, treat both the inside and outside entry points.

3. At night, after the ants have gone back to their nest, apply the lavender essential oil to each entry point. Repeat twice daily until the ants stop looking for a way inside your home.

## Peppermint-Tea Tree Ant Spray

Makes about 4 ounces

Peppermint, tea tree, and lavender are natural ant repellants. While this spray won't kill them, it can prevent them from staying in your home. For best results, treat countertops, sinks, garbage cans, windowsills, and doorframes with this spray.

2 ounces distilled water
2 ounces rubbing alcohol
20 drops peppermint essential oil
15 drops tea tree essential oil
8 drops lavender essential oil

1. In a bottle with a fine-mist spray top, combine all the ingredients. Shake well to blend, and then shake again before each use.

2. Spray a fine mist onto areas where ant activity has been noticed. Repeat two to three times daily until ant activity stops.

## Peppermint Ant Killer

Makes about 6 ounces

Peppermint essential oil combines with old-fashioned blue dish soap, to kill and repel ants.

2 ounces blue dish soap
4 ounces distilled water
30 drops peppermint essential oil

1. In a bottle with a trigger spray top, combine all the ingredients. Shake well to blend, and then shake again before each use.

2. Spray any ants you see with the solution; they will die immediately. Wipe up dead ants with a paper towel and discard it.

3. Spray the spaces of your home where the ants are entering, but do not wipe it up. Check every few hours for dead ants and wipe them up. Repeat the treatment two to three times daily until ant activity stops.

# BATHROOM CLEANSERS

Store-bought bathroom cleaners often have a strong antiseptic smell, but it doesn't have to be that way. Aromatherapy-based cleansers can transform your bathroom into a squeaky clean spa-like environment. And, as a bonus, there are no nasty chemicals.

## All-Purpose Disinfectant Spray

*Makes about 9 ounces*

Lemon, sweet orange and tea tree kill bacteria without the toxicity of regular cleaners. This fantastic all-purpose bathroom spray keeps surfaces sparkly and makes daily cleanups enjoyable. This spray is ideal for the bathtub, toilet, sink, tile, and hard-surface floors.

1 cup distilled water
1 teaspoon baking soda
1 tablespoon liquid castile soap
15 drops tea tree essential oil
10 drops sweet orange essential oil
5 drops lemon essential oil

1. In a bottle with a trigger spray top, combine the water and baking soda, and then shake to blend.

2. Add the castile soap and swirl the bottle to blend it in, and then add the essential oils. Shake well to blend, and then shake again before each use.

3. Apply 1 spritz to each area you'd like to address, using a spritz or more if needed. Wipe clean with a paper towel or cloth. Use as often as needed.

## Lemon Scouring Powder

*Makes 8 ounces*

Lemon essential oil kills germs and combines with borax to gently scrub your toilet bowl clean without exposing you to harmful fumes found in traditional cleaners.

1 cup borax
12 drops lemon essential oil

1. In a sugar shaker, combine the borax with the lemon essential oil, using a fork to stir.

2. Turn off the toilet's water supply, and then flush the toilet. Sprinkle the bowl with a dusting of scouring powder, and then use a toilet brush to scrub thoroughly.

3. Turn the water supply back on. After the tank fills, flush the toilet.

## Daily Tea Tree-Eucalyptus Shower Spray

*Makes about 8 ounces*

Tea tree and eucalyptus inhibit mold growth, keeping your shower sanitary while preventing you from having to deep clean it quite so often.

3½ cups distilled water
½ cup rubbing alcohol
20 drops tea tree essential oil
10 drops eucalyptus essential oil

1. In a bottle with a trigger spray top, combine all the ingredients. Shake well to blend, and then shake again before each use.

2. After every shower, mist the walls, floors, and shower curtain or door, making sure to coat all surfaces. Pay special attention to areas where water tends to collect. Repeat daily.

**PREFERENCE TIP** If you'd like a softer scent, try a combination of 20 drops of lavender and 10 drops of lemon instead of the tea tree–eucalyptus combo in this recipe.

# DISHES

It takes a little bit of effort to keep your dishes clean and sparkling, but when you add aromatherapy into the mix, your daily dishwashing tasks will seem a little less difficult and certainly more fragrant.

## Liquid Lavender Dish Soap

Makes about 16 ounces

Lavender essential oil and a few simple ingredients get dishes clean while treating you to a pleasant, chemical-free fragrance. Inhale deeply while washing your dishes for a pleasurable experience.

**1 tablespoon castile bar soap, grated**
**1 tablespoon borax**
**1¾ cups boiling water**
**32 drops lavender essential oil**

1. In a large bowl, combine the grated bar soap and the borax. Whisk to blend thoroughly, and then add the boiling water.

2. Continue whisking carefully until the grated soap melts completely. Allow the mixture to cool, and then add the essential oil. Whisk again.

3. Transfer the blend to a plastic squeeze bottle or a bottle with a pump top. A pre-used, sanitized dish soap bottle is ideal.

4. The mixture will thicken into a gel within 6 to 8 hours. Then use as you would any dish soap.

SUBSTITUTION TIP For a perkier citrus version, substitute the lavender with 8 drops of lemon essential oil and 12 drops of mandarin essential oil.

## Lemon Dishwasher Detergent

Makes 4 cups

Lemon, washing soda, and borax get dishes clean and leave your dishwasher smelling fresh, minus the toxic, environmentally unsustainable chemicals found in most commercial dishwasher detergents.

2 cups washing soda
2 cups borax
16 drops lemon essential oil

1. In a blender or food processor, combine all the ingredients. Process on the lowest speed until the washing soda crystals have been reduced to powder.

2. Allow the dust inside the blender or food processor to settle before opening the lid, and then transfer the powder to a large, sealed container.

3. Load your dishwasher and add 2 tablespoons of powder to the detergent compartment. Use a little more or less as needed, and run your dishwasher as usual.

PREFERENCE TIP If you'd like to eliminate chemical-laden rinse aids as well, fill the rinse-aid compartment with white vinegar and a few drops of lemon essential oil.

## Lemon-Tea Tree Dishwasher Pods

Makes about 30 pods

Lemon and tea tree sanitize dishes, and simple soap ingredients save you money while being safe for your family and the environment.

2 cups borax
2 cups baking soda
½ cup Epsom salt
½ cup white vinegar
12 drops lemon essential oil
12 drops tea tree essential oil

1. In a large bowl, combine all the ingredients using a wooden spoon. A lumpy consistency is normal.

2. Pack the mixture tightly into 2 ice cube trays, ensuring that the finished product will fit into your dishwasher's soap compartment. Place the filled molds in a warm, dry spot for 48 hours and then transfer to a large jar or plastic food storage container.

3. Add one pod to the dishwasher's soap compartment, close the lid, and run your dishwasher as usual.

PREFERENCE TIP If you're tired of cloudy-looking glassware from hard water, add ½ cup of white vinegar to the bottom of your dishwasher before each load.

# FLEAS

Dogs and cats enrich our lives, but when they attract fleas, or worse become infested, discomfort and even disease can result. Before reaching for chemical flea treatments, give these simple, all-natural solutions a try.

## Lavender Flea Powder

Makes 1 ounce

Lavender essential oil is safe for cats and dogs, and it repels fleas. Baking soda damages the exoskeletons of the fleas and kills them, plus it soothes your pet's itchy skin. Use this remedy in conjunction with Indoor Flea Powder (page 299), and wash your pet's bedding in hot, soapy water before applying the flea powder.

1 cup baking soda
12 drops lavender essential oil for dogs;
   1 drop lavender essential oil for cats

1. In a large measuring cup, use a fork to stir the lavender essential oil into the baking soda. Sift the blend into a bowl to remove any lumps, and then transfer it to a glass or metal sugar shaker.

2. To use on dogs, apply a light dusting of powder along the dog's back and then work it into the fur with your fingers. Have your dog roll over and repeat the process on the underside.

3. To use on cats, sprinkle about ½ teaspoon of powder onto the palm of your hand, and then gently stroke your cat's fur, being sure to avoid the eye area.

4. Wait 3 to 4 hours, and then use a flea comb to remove dead and dying fleas. Repeat weekly during flea season.

## Synergistic Dog Flea Collar Blend

Makes 1 ounce

A powerful combination of citronella, cedar, rosemary, and peppermint essential oils kills and repels fleas for up to a month. This blend is only safe for dogs; do not use this blend or any of these essential oils on cats or other small animals. Also, be sure to check your dog for sensitivity 1 hour after applying the collar and 24 hours later. If you notice irritation, remove the collar and try Lavender Flea Powder (page 298) instead.

2 teaspoons citronella essential oil
2 teaspoons rosemary essential oil
1 teaspoon Atlas cedarwood essential oil
1 teaspoon peppermint essential oil
1 cotton dog collar in your dog's size

1. In a small bottle with an orifice reducer, combine all the essential oils. Shake well to blend, and allow the blend to rest for 24 hours before use.

2. Apply the blend directly to the underside of the collar, which will come into contact with your dog's skin. For dogs under 30 pounds, use 6 drops. For dogs over 30 pounds, use 10 drops.

3. Remove the collar each time the dog bathes or swims. Reapply the blend to the collar every 1 to 4 weeks.

## Indoor Flea Powder

Makes 16 ounces

Lavender essential oil, borax, and salt combine to kill fleas and their eggs inside your home. For outdoor use, replace the salt with diatomaceous earth to avoid harming plants. This remedy is not for use on your pets.

12 ounces borax
4 ounces salt
8 drops lavender essential oil
1 teaspoon of uncooked rice
  (optional, for humidity control)

1. In a large bowl, combine all the ingredients. Whisk to blend thoroughly. If you are in a humid climate, add the rice to keep the powder from clumping, and mix in well. Transfer the powder to a glass or metal sugar shaker.

2. Sprinkle the powder liberally throughout your home. Use a stiff broom to work the powder deep into carpeting or area rugs. On non-carpeted floors, use the broom to work the powder into all the crevices. Leave the treatment in place for 2 days.

3. After 2 days, wash all of your pet's bedding in very hot, soapy water to kill any fleas that may be hiding there. Then, thoroughly vacuum all areas throughout your home.

4. Repeat this treatment once weekly during a heavy infestation; for a light infestation, one treatment should be enough.

# FLOORS

With proper maintenance, your floors will look beautiful for many years. Instead of spending a fortune on expensive, toxic cleaning solutions, reach for these fragrant, all-natural floor cleaners.

## Mandarin-Neroli Carpet Powder

Makes about 8 ounces

Mandarin and neroli combine with a hint of ginger and powerful baking soda to knock out odors and give your home a fresh, irresistible fragrance that's sure to boost your mood.

8 ounces baking soda
20 drops mandarin essential oil
8 drops neroli essential oil
3 drops ginger essential oil
1 teaspoon of uncooked rice
   (optional, for humidity control)

1. In a large bowl, combine all the ingredients. Whisk to blend thoroughly. If you are in a humid climate, add the rice to keep the powder from clumping, and mix in well. Transfer the powder to a glass or metal sugar shaker.

2. Sprinkle a light dusting of powder onto carpets and area rugs. Allow the blend to remain in place for 10 minutes to 1 hour, and then vacuum it up. Repeat as often as you like.

PREFERENCE TIP You can use any of your favorite aromatherapy blends to create a carpet powder that appeals to you, so feel free to experiment with different oils.

## Lavender-Eucalyptus Mop Solution

Makes 1 treatment

Lavender and eucalyptus sanitize your floors, while vinegar and baking soda combine with a little bit of liquid dish soap to remove dirt and leave surfaces clean and shiny. This solution is best for tile and linoleum floors.

2 gallons hot tap water
1 cup baking soda
1 cup white vinegar
2 teaspoons liquid dish soap
8 drops lavender essential oil
4 drops eucalyptus essential oil (any species)

1. In a mop bucket, combine all the ingredients. Swish the mop through the mixture to blend.

2. Mop the floor as usual, occasionally rinsing the dirt from your mop in a bucket of clear water before dipping it back into the solution.

SUBSTITUTION TIP For laminate floors, use 2 cups of water, 1 tablespoon of vinegar, 1 tablespoon of baking soda, and 4 drops of your favorite essential oil in a spray bottle. Spritz floors before using a dry mop or apply to a Swiffer-type pad.

## Citrus Hardwood Floor Cleaner

Makes 8 ounces

With fragrant mandarin and grapefruit essential oils, this solution cuts through dirt, leaving hardwood floors sparkling while promoting a happy, carefree mood.

7 ounces distilled water
1 ounce white vinegar
2 drops liquid dish detergent
4 drops grapefruit essential oil
2 drops mandarin essential oil

1. In a bottle with a fine-mist spray top, combine all the ingredients. Shake well to blend, and then shake again before each use.

2. Apply a light mist of the solution to the floor, and then mop with a dry mop. Work in two- to four-foot sections to prevent the solution from evaporating before you arrive with the mop. Repeat two to three times weekly, or as often as needed.

# GLASS AND MIRRORS

Clean, sparkling windows and mirrors make your home a more pleasant place to be. Try these fragrant solutions instead of reaching for expensive sprays that might contain toxic ingredients.

## Lemon Window Cleaner

Makes about 16 ounces

Lemon essential oil, rubbing alcohol, and vinegar remove smudges from windows quickly. It's also ideal for glass tabletops.

1 cup water
1 cup rubbing alcohol
1 tablespoon white vinegar
6 drops lemon essential oil

1. In a bottle with a trigger spray top, combine all the ingredients. Shake well to blend, and then shake again before each use.

2. Spray the blend onto the window, and then wipe clean with a rag or a paper towel. Repeat as needed.

## Heavy-Duty Window Cleaner

Makes about 16 ounces

Tea tree essential oil and simple ingredients like vinegar and dish soap make a strong window cleaner that removes heavy layers of grime or pollen. This is ideal for the exterior side of the window, as well as for grimy glass doors.

8 ounces vinegar
8 ounces warm water
½ teaspoon liquid dish detergent
8 drops tea tree essential oil

1. In a bottle with a trigger spray top, combine all the ingredients. Shake well to blend, and then shake again before each use.

2. Spray the blend onto the window, and then wipe clean with a rag or a paper towel. Repeat as needed.

## Streak-Free Glass and Mirror Cleaner

Makes about 10 ounces

Lemon eucalyptus kills bacteria and imparts a light, fresh scent to this simple streak-free cleaner.

1 cup distilled water
1 ounce rubbing alcohol
1 ounce white vinegar
1½ teaspoons cornstarch
12 drops lemon eucalyptus essential oil

1. In a bottle with a trigger spray top, combine all the ingredients. Shake well to blend, and then shake again before each use.

2. Spray the blend onto the window, and then wipe clean with a rag or a paper towel. Repeat as needed.

# GYM BAGS AND SPORTS EQUIPMENT

Fitness is an important part of natural health, but it's hard to enjoy the gym when your gear has a funky smell. Mild, fragrant aromatherapy solutions offer a fantastic, nontoxic alternative to harsh chemical cleaners.

## Gym Bag Freshener

Makes about 4 ounces

Tea tree essential oil kills the fungus and bacteria that's behind the dreaded gym bag odor. After an initial deep cleaning, weekly maintenance will keep your bag smelling its best. It also helps to avoid leaving soiled items in the bag overnight.

2 ounces distilled water
2 ounces rubbing alcohol
16 drops tea tree essential oil

1. Remove everything from your gym bag, including the removable plastic piece at the bottom, if any. Wash and dry a heavily soiled gym bag before using the freshener.

2. In a bottle with a trigger spray top, combine all the ingredients. Shake well to blend, and then shake again before each use.

3. Apply a fine mist of the freshener to the entire gym bag, inside and out, including the plastic parts and inside the pockets.

4. Allow the bag to dry completely before repacking it. Repeat once weekly.

## Shoe, Glove, and Helmet Spray

Makes about 8 ounces

Lemon and clove bud kill bacteria and leave a pleasant, invigorating scent behind. Use this spray to keep shoes, gloves, helmets, football pads, jock straps, and other sporting goods smelling fresh between uses. If items are heavily soiled, wash them according to the manufacturer's instructions before using this spray.

4 ounces distilled water
4 ounces rubbing alcohol
20 drops clove bud essential oil
20 drops lemon essential oil

1. In a bottle with a fine-mist spray top, combine all the ingredients. Shake well to blend, and then shake again before each use.

2. Apply a fine mist of spray to the item requiring cleansing, and then wipe down with a soft cloth or a paper towel. If you won't be using the item immediately, apply a second fine mist and allow it to air-dry. Repeat as needed.

## Bay Laurel Yoga Mat Spray

Makes about 4 ounces

Bay laurel essential oil kills bacteria and fungi, plus its fragrance enhances focus.

4 ounces alcohol-free witch hazel
12 drops bay laurel essential oil

1. In a bottle with a fine-mist spray top, combine all the ingredients. Shake well to blend, and then shake again before each use.

2. If your yoga mat is heavily soiled, give it a good wipe down with mild soap and water, and then rinse it. Allow it to air-dry before moving to the next step.

3. Apply a fine mist of spray to the entire yoga mat, and repeat immediately after each use. If you have time, let it air-dry before you roll it up. Repeat as needed.

PREFERENCE TIP If you prefer a different fragrance, feel free to try others, such as lemon, lavender, or clove bud essential oil in place of the bay laurel.

# KITCHEN CLEANSERS

Foodborne illness is a real threat, so it's important to keep your kitchen clean. Luckily, you can accomplish this task without relying on toxic commercial solutions.

## Quick Countertop Wipes

Makes 80 to 100 disposable wipes

Lemon, rosemary, and tea tree kill germs, while castile soap is gentle on delicate surfaces. These wipes are safe for all countertops, including granite and marble ones.

1 roll premium paper towels
1 cup distilled water
1 cup rubbing alcohol
1 tablespoon liquid castile soap
10 drops lemon essential oil
10 drops rosemary essential oil
10 drops tea tree essential oils

1. With a sharp plain-edge knife, cut the paper towel roll in half horizontally.

2. In a large bowl, combine all the ingredients. Stir well.

3. Place one half of the paper towel roll into the bowl, allowing the roll to absorb some of the liquid. Flip the roll over to ensure even absorption. Repeat the process with the other half of the paper towel roll.

4. Pull the cardboard cores out of the center of each roll to allow you to pull wipes up from the center. Place each roll of wipes in a one-gallon plastic zip-top bag. (Plastic food storage containers also work well.)

5. Use wipes as needed to clean up spills or just spruce up your countertops.

## Microwave Disinfectant

Makes 1 treatment

Clean and disinfect your microwave without spending any time scrubbing. Lemon provides a fresh, clean scent.

1 cup hot tap water
1 cup vinegar
1 drop lemon essential oil

1. In a microwave-safe bowl, combine all the ingredients. Place the bowl in the microwave and run on high power for 5 to 10 minutes.

2. With oven mitts, remove the bowl from the microwave and discard the solution. Wipe down the interior of the microwave with paper towels or a rag. Repeat as needed.

## Oven/Stovetop Gentle Scrubbing Soap

Makes 12 ounces

Sweet orange and clove bud essential oils kill bacteria, and baking soda makes short work of grime. This blend is fantastic for ovens, stovetops, and sinks, and it's great for bathtubs and showers, too. It will keep your appliances looking sparkly inside and out.

1 cup baking soda
2 tablespoons castile soap
2 tablespoons distilled water
12 drops sweet orange essential oil
4 drops clove bud essential oil
2 tablespoons vinegar

1. In a large bowl, combine the baking soda and castile soap. Stir well to blend. Add the water and essential oils, and stir again.

2. Add the vinegar slowly. It is normal for the mixture to produce bubbles. Stir again until well combined. If the mixture is thicker than desired, add a little more water, 1 teaspoon at a time. Transfer the scrub to a plastic squeeze bottle.

3. Apply 1 teaspoon of the soft scrub to a sponge, moisten the area to be cleaned, and scrub. Rinse with water when finished. Repeat as needed.

# LAUNDRY

Commercial laundry soaps often contain toxins, as well as phosphorus, which is bad for the planet and your skin. Homemade aromatherapy laundry solutions get your clothes clean, while making laundry day a much more enjoyable experience.

## May Chang Laundry Detergent

Makes enough for 80 loads

May Chang essential oil kills bacteria and infuses laundry with an intriguing citrus scent.

2 bars castile soap, grated
2 cups baking soda
2 cups washing soda
1 cup kosher salt
20 drops May Chang essential oil

1. In a food processor or blender, combine the castile soap, baking soda, washing soda, and salt. Pulse until the castile soap shreds have been combined with the rest of the blend. Alternatively, whisk the blend thoroughly to combine the ingredients.

2. Add the essential oil to the mixture a few drops at a time, stirring after each addition. Transfer the finished laundry detergent to a large jar or canister.

3. Use 1 tablespoon per load of laundry. If you have a large-capacity machine that handles double or triple loads, use 2 to 3 tablespoons per cycle.

SUBSTITUTION TIP If you don't have May Chang essential oil, feel free to be creative with your choice of oil. Lemon, spearmint, and patchouli are interesting alternatives, and lavender always works well.

## Lavender Fabric Softener

Makes enough for about 32 loads

Lavender makes laundry smell fantastic, and Epsom salt leaves clothing feeling silky soft.

**4 cups Epsom salt**
**10 drops lavender essential oil**

1. In a large bowl, combine the ingredients. Whisk to blend thoroughly, and then transfer to a large jar or canister.

2. After loading the laundry into the washing machine, sprinkle 2 tablespoons of fabric softener on top and run the machine as usual. If you have a large-capacity machine that handles double or triple loads, use 4 to 6 tablespoons per cycle.

PREFERENCE TIP If you'd prefer a more natural fabric softener sheet than those you find on your store shelves, add 4 to 6 drops of your favorite essential oil to a damp washcloth and toss it in the dryer with your damp clothing.

## Aromatherapy Dryer Sheet

Makes 1 reusable dryer sheet

Essential oils give your laundry a lovely fragrance. When combined with the Lavender Fabric Softener, this reusable dryer sheet eliminates the need for disposable ones.

**1 clean washcloth**
**10 drops essential oil or blend, your choice**

1. Apply the essential oil or blend to the washcloth and toss it in the dryer along with your damp laundry.

2. Run the dryer as usual. Your clothes will emerge with a fresh, natural scent.

# LAWN AND GARDEN

Chemical herbicides and pesticides are expensive, and they aren't the best choices for the planet or your homegrown vegetables. Try these gentle, earth-friendly options instead.

## Cinnamon Leaf Weed Killer

Makes about 8 ounces

Cinnamon leaf essential oil contains a chemical called *eugenol,* which is a strong natural weed killer. This remedy works best on young weeds; however, you can chop the tops off older weeds and apply it to the freshly cut area.

**4 ounces sunflower oil**
**4 ounces white vinegar**
**40 drops cinnamon leaf essential oil**

1. In a bottle with a trigger spray top, combine all the ingredients. Shake well to blend, and then shake again before each use.

2. Choose a calm, sunny day to apply the weed killer, and head out to the garden as soon as any dew dries so that the oil will have all day to work.

3. Spray the center growing tip as well as the leaves of each weed you want to kill. Repeat whenever weeds reemerge.

SUBSTITUTION TIP If you don't have cinnamon leaf essential oil, you can try pine, clove bud, or thyme instead.

## Slug and Snail Repellent

Makes about 8 ounces

Slugs and snails are sensitive creatures, and pine essential oil drives them away from tender plants.

**16 jar lids or small, flat containers**
**8 ounces water**
**20 drops pine essential oil**

1. In a bottle, combine the ingredients. Shake well to blend.

2. Set the containers around your garden, especially near plants that tend to attract slugs and snails. Pour 1 tablespoon of the blend into each one.

3. Check the lids periodically to ensure that they still smell like pine. Replace the repellent when the scent fades. Repeat the process as needed.

## Tea Tree Antifungal Plant Treatment

Makes 1 gallon

Tea tree essential oil is a powerful antifungal agent that prevents fungus from attacking and killing your plants. Powdery mildew, blight, rust, and other common garden fungi are no match for it. Choose a mild, preferably overcast day for the treatment, or treat plants in the evening to prevent sunburn.

**1 gallon water**
**12 drops tea tree essential oil**

1. In a clean garden pump sprayer that has never held herbicide, combine the ingredients. Shake vigorously to blend.

2. Operate the pump sprayer according to its manufacturer's instructions, and apply a fine mist to all affected plants as well as any that might be susceptible to fungus.

# LEATHER CARE

Like your skin, leather requires special care. Because some leather items are treated with protective or decorative coatings, it's important to test these solutions in an inconspicuous area before applying them to the entire item.

## Elemi Leather Cleaner

Makes 4 ounces

Elemi softens and protects leather, while castile soap and vinegar clean it gently.

3 ounces white vinegar
1 ounce liquid castile soap
4 drops elemi essential oil

1. In a bottle or jar, combine all the ingredients. Shake well to blend, and then shake again before each use.

2. With a clean rag or sponge, apply ½ teaspoon of the blend to the item you'd like to clean. Gently rub it in, using small, circular motions. Use a little more or less as needed.

3. With a second cloth or sponge, wipe the item dry. Repeat as needed.

## Lemon Conditioning Balm

Makes about 4 ounces

Lemon essential oil is fantastic for leather, as it prevents cracking and dryness.

1 ounce beeswax, melted
1 ounce cocoa butter, melted
2 ounces sweet almond oil
40 drops lemon essential oil

1. In a medium bowl, combine all the ingredients. Whisk to blend thoroughly, and then transfer the balm to a jar.

2. With a soft cloth, apply ½ teaspoon of the blend to the item you'd like to condition. Use small, circular motions to work the conditioner into the leather.

3. When finished, buff the leather with a clean cloth to bring out the shine. Repeat as needed.

## Tea Tree Mildew Treatment

Makes 1 treatment

If a leather item has been damaged by mildew, don't despair. Tea tree essential oil will get rid of the fungus, and as long as the leather isn't badly cracked or rotted, you can use conditioning balm to restore it.

1 tablespoon white vinegar
4 drops tea tree essential oil

1. With a soft cloth or a soft-bristled brush, apply the vinegar and scrub the mildew off the item.

2. Wipe away the vinegar and mildew, and then use a second cloth or brush to apply the essential oil. Use a little more or less as needed, ensuring you cover the area where the mildew was present.

3. Allow the leather to dry, and then apply the Lemon Conditioning Balm. Check the item in 1 week to see if it still has a mildew odor. If so, repeat the treatment.

# LINENS

Fresh linens—tablecloths, napkins, towels, and sheets—are essential to everyday life. Fragrant aromatherapy solutions make using them a special treat.

## Aromatherapy Ironing Spray

Makes 8 ounces

Lavender, clary sage, and neroli create a delightful fragrance that puts your mind at ease and helps you look forward to getting the wrinkles out of linens and clothing.

8 ounces distilled water
8 drops clary sage essential oil
8 drops lavender essential oil
2 drops neroli essential oil

1. In a bottle with a fine-mist spray top, combine all the ingredients. Shake well to blend, and then shake again before each use.

2. Apply a spritz to the area you're about to iron. Repeat as needed.

## Bergamot-Cedarwood Sachets

Makes 4 sachets

Bergamot and cedarwood give linens an inviting scent while preventing mustiness and keeping bugs out of storage areas.

1 cup baking soda
12 drops bergamot essential oil
24 drops cedarwood essential oil
4 (3 x 5-inch) muslin sachet bags

1. In a medium bowl, combine all the ingredients. Whisk to blend thoroughly. Sift the mixture into a second bowl to eliminate any lumps.

2. With a funnel, carefully transfer ¼ cup of the blend into each of the sachet bags. Tighten the drawstrings, and place the bags in your linen closet or drawers.

3. When the scent fades, add 3 drops of bergamot and 6 drops of cedarwood essential oil to the powder inside the bag and stir with a thin utensil.

STORAGE Keep in areas where linens are stored.

## Lavender Dryer Balls

Makes 1 set of dryer balls

Skip the expensive dryer balls and grab a tube of brand-new tennis balls. These, along with lavender essential oil, will fluff your linens and leave them smelling fantastic.

8 drops lavender essential oil
4 brand-new tennis balls

1. Apply 2 drops of lavender essential oil to each tennis ball. Transfer the balls to a canister or storage container.

2. When fluffing or drying linens, place all 4 balls in the dryer. Run the dryer as usual, listening carefully for the cycle to end. Immediately remove the linens from the dryer and dress the bed, table, or bathroom towel bars.

3. When the scent fades from the balls, add another 2 drops of lavender essential oil to each ball.

# MOLD AND MILDEW

Mold and mildew grow best in dark, damp places. Essential oils work wonders for prevention as well as for cleanups. For major issues, it's best to contact a mold remediation expert.

## Mold and Mildew Prevention Spray

Makes 8 ounces

Tea tree and lemon essential oils kill mold and mildew spores in areas where they tend to grow. This spray is ideal for kitchen and bath use.

3 ounces white vinegar
5 ounces distilled water
6 drops tea tree essential oil
4 drops lemon essential oil
2 drops clove bud essential oil

1. In a bottle with a fine-mist spray top, combine all the ingredients. Shake well to blend, and then shake again before each use.

2. Apply 1 to 2 spritzes to each area where mold and mildew tend to appear.

3. Allow the area to air-dry. Repeat once weekly, and increase use to twice per week in warm, damp spaces or during periods of muggy weather.

## Tea Tree Mold Remover

Makes 1 ounce

Tea tree essential oil kills tough mold, like the kind that can show up on grout, wooden backsplashes, and other vulnerable areas.

½ ounce tea tree essential oil
½ ounce distilled water

1. In a small bottle with an orifice reducer, combine the ingredients. Shake well to blend, and then shake again before each use.

2. Apply 1 drop to each area of mold that you'd like to address, using a little more if needed and making sure to cover the entire moldy area.

3. Allow to air-dry. Repeat as needed to stop moldy patches from forming.

## Tea Tree Wall Mold Diffusion

Makes 1 treatment

Painted walls and bare wood often attract mold during muggy weather, even when the rest of your home is spotless. Diffusing tea tree essential oil next to the affected area kills the mold and prevents its return.

10 drops tea tree essential oil

1. Remove pets and children under 12 years from the room requiring treatment.

2. Add the essential oil to your diffuser according to the manufacturer's instructions. Run the diffuser for 1 hour within a foot of the moldy area, positioning it so that the diffused oil will contact the affected surface.

3. Leave the moldy area alone for 24 hours, and then wipe the area with a paper towel, working from the mold's outer edge toward its center. If any stubborn mold remains, repeat the process.

PREGNANCY-FRIENDLY TIP If you are pregnant or nursing, leave the room while the diffuser is running. It's okay to go back in to shut the diffuser off, but like young children and pets, it's best for you to stay out of the room for as long as the tea tree aroma is strong.

# MOSQUITOES

Mosquitoes, gnats, chiggers, and other insects can ruin outdoor fun fast. Fragrant aromatherapy treatments keep biting insects at bay and eliminate the need for toxic insect repellents.

## Mosquito Repellent Spray

Makes about 8 ounces

Mosquitoes can't stand citronella or eucalyptus, and lemon is a strong deterrent as well.

4 ounces distilled water
4 ounces unflavored vodka
40 drops citronella essential oil
20 drops *Eucalyptus radiata* essential oil
10 drops lemon essential oil

1. In a bottle with a fine-mist spray top, combine all the ingredients. Shake well to blend, and then shake again before each use.

2. Apply 1 spritz to each area of exposed skin. When insect activity is high, use the spray on clothing, hats, and other items such as outdoor canopies and camping tents.

SUBSTITUTION TIP If you don't have *Eucalyptus radiata*, feel free to use *Eucalyptus globulus* or lemon eucalyptus in its place.

## Mason Jar Luminaries

Makes 3 luminaries

Rosemary, lemon, cedarwood, and lavender combine with citronella to keep bugs from spoiling alfresco dining experiences. Add fresh herbs and citrus slices to create beautiful, natural decorations for your table.

3 (8-ounce) mason jars
30 drops cedarwood essential oil
30 drops citronella essential oil
30 drops lavender essential oil
30 drops lemon essential oil
30 drops rosemary essential oil
6 sprigs fresh rosemary, lavender, or basil
1 lemon, thinly sliced
1 lime, thinly sliced
24 ounces tap water
3 floating tea lights

1. Into the bottom of each jar, place 10 drops of each of the essential oils.

2. Insert two sprigs of the herb into each of the jars, bending the stems as needed to keep the tops from poking out.

3. Divide the lemon and lime slices among the jars and layer them on top of the herbs.

4. Fill each jar with the water to just below its neck, and then float a tea light on top of the water.

5. Arrange the luminaries on the table and light the candles. Enjoy! Discard the contents after a day or so.

## Patchouli-Spearmint Repellent Lotion

Makes about 8 ounces

Patchouli, spearmint, and lavender repel biting bugs, while the lotion leaves skin feeling smooth and soft.

8 ounces unscented body lotion
   or hand cream
20 drops patchouli essential oil
10 drops lavender essential oil
10 drops spearmint essential oil

1. In a large bowl, combine all the ingredients. Whisk to blend thoroughly, and then transfer the lotion to a jar or back to its original container.

2. Apply 1 teaspoon of the lotion to exposed skin. Use a little more or less as needed, and feel free to apply the lotion to body parts that are covered. The more fragrant you are, the less biting bugs will like you! Repeat as needed.

STORAGE Keep this lotion in a convenient location if you plan to use it all within two weeks; otherwise, keep it in a glass bottle or jar in a cool, dark place.

# MOTHS

Given the opportunity, moths will get into linen closets, cupboards, and pantries, where they feed and reproduce. These preventives are safe, all-natural alternatives to toxic mothballs and insecticides.

## Pantry Moth Repellent

Makes about 4 ounces

Bay laurel and lavender combine with lemon, eucalyptus, and peppermint to keep pantry moths from invading dry foodstuffs. Remember to seal dried goods in airtight containers if pantry moths are a problem in your area.

4 ounces vinegar
40 drops bay laurel essential oil
40 drops *Eucalyptus globulus* essential oil
20 drops lavender essential oil
20 drops lemon essential oil
10 drops peppermint essential oil

1. In a bottle with a fine-mist spray top, combine all the ingredients. Shake well to blend, and then shake again before each use.

2. Clear the pantry of all food and wash shelves with soap and water. Allow the area to air-dry, and then apply a fine mist of the spray to shelves and walls, paying special attention to cracks and crevices. The solution will prevent any moth eggs from hatching. Repeat every 2 to 3 months to prevent reinfestation.

## Citronella-Lavender Mothballs

Makes 20 moth balls

Citronella and lavender discourage moths from entering their favorite hiding spaces. These simple mothballs are nontoxic and leave your home smelling fresh.

20 cotton balls
40 drops citronella essential oil
40 drops lavender essential oil

1. On each cotton ball, apply 2 drops of citronella and 2 drops of lavender essential oil.
2. Place the mothballs in cabinets, drawers, and other areas where moth activity has been problematic. Refresh the mothballs with more essential oil every 2 to 4 weeks, or when you notice the scent has faded.

## Patchouli-Palo Santo Potpourri

Makes 4 cups

Patchouli and palo santo essential oils repel moths, and combine beautifully with cedar chips. A jar of potpourri adds fragrance to your closet while deterring pesky bugs.

4 cups cedar chips
40 drops palo santo essential oil
40 drops patchouli essential oil
4 (8-ounce) jars

1. Place the cedar chips in a large bowl. Add the essential oils 4 to 5 drops at a time, stirring with a spatula between additions. Divide the potpourri among the four jars.
2. Place the jars uncovered in the back corners of closets or wardrobes. Refresh the potpourri with more essential oils when the scent fades.

# OUTDOOR FURNITURE

Outdoor living spaces add beauty and value to your home. It's easy to use aromatherapy-based cleaners to freshen and maintain the furnishings that help you enjoy these special spaces.

## Lemon-Citronella Wicker Balm

Makes about 8 ounces

Wicker furniture is easy to rinse off with a hose. Once you've removed dirt, use this balm to add a layer of protection from insects and moisture, and to impart a light, pleasant aroma.

4 ounces sweet almond oil
2 ounces beeswax, melted
2 ounces cocoa butter, melted
40 drops citronella essential oil
40 drops lemon essential oil

1. In a medium bowl, combine all the ingredients. Whisk to blend thoroughly, and then transfer the balm to a jar.

2. With a soft cloth, apply ½ teaspoon of the blend to the wicker item. Use small, circular motions to work the conditioner into the wicker.

3. When finished, buff the wicker with a clean cloth to bring out the shine. Repeat as needed.

## Lemon Wood Conditioner

Makes about 4 ounces

Lemon essential oil combines with sweet almond oil to moisturize and protect wood furniture. This treatment isn't meant for teak furniture, and it causes some types of wood to darken. Test it in an inconspicuous spot before conditioning the entire item.

4 ounces sweet almond oil
40 drops lemon essential oil

1. In a bottle or jar, combine the ingredients. Shake well to blend.

2. With a soft cloth, apply ¼ teaspoon of the oil to the item. Rub in small, circular motions and add more conditioner as needed until the entire item has been treated.

3. When finished, buff the wood with a clean cloth to bring out the shine. Repeat as needed.

## Citrus-Clove Bud Outdoor Upholstery Spray

Makes about 8 ounces

Lemon, clove bud, and sweet orange refresh outdoor upholstery and prevent mildew. Add another layer of protection to cushions and other fabric items by covering them or storing them in a sheltered area when precipitation is in the forecast.

4 ounces filtered water
4 ounces rubbing alcohol
20 drops clove bud essential oil
20 drops lemon essential oil
20 drops sweet orange essential oil

1. In a bottle with a fine-mist spray top, combine all the ingredients. Shake well to blend, and then shake again before each use.

2. Apply a light mist of spray onto each item so that all areas are covered. Allow items to air-dry before use. Repeat as needed.

# PET ODOR

Pets are wonderful companions—even if they tend to leave odors behind. Aromatherapy can keep a home with furry creatures smelling fresh around the clock, eliminating the needs for toxic chemical deodorants.

## Lavender Litter Box Deodorizer

*Makes 8 ounces*

Lavender kills bacteria, while baking soda makes short work of tough odors. Clean litter boxes daily for best results.

**8 ounces baking soda**
**2 drops lavender essential oil**
**1 teaspoon uncooked rice**
    **(optional, for humidity control)**

1. In a large bowl, combine the ingredients. Stir well to blend.

2. Sift the blend into a second bowl to eliminate lumps. If you are in a humid climate, add the rice to keep the powder from clumping, and mix in well. Transfer the mixture to a glass or metal sugar shaker.

3. Sprinkle 1 to 2 tablespoons of the deodorizer onto the surface of the freshly cleaned litter. Repeat each time you clean the litter box.

## Doggie Bed Freshening Spray

Makes about 8 ounces

Lavender and tea tree combine to keep your dog's bed smelling fresh and clean between washes. Do not use this spray on cat beds.

4 ounces distilled water
4 ounces rubbing alcohol
20 drops lavender essential oil
10 drops tea tree essential oil

1. In a bottle with a fine-mist spray top, combine all the ingredients. Shake well to blend, and then shake again before each use.

2. Apply 1 to 3 spritzes to your dog's bedding, ensuring that you've covered the entire surface. Use a little more if you have a very large pet.

## Lavender Carpet Powder

Makes 8 ounces

Lavender and baking soda deodorize carpets fast, and as a bonus, this blend costs far less than commercial carpet powders.

1 cup baking soda
12 drops lavender essential oil
1 teaspoon of uncooked rice
    (optional, for humidity control)

1. In a large bowl, combine the ingredients. Stir well to blend.

2. Sift the blend into a second bowl to eliminate lumps. If you are in a humid climate, add the rice to keep the powder from clumping, and mix in well. Transfer the mixture to a glass or metal sugar shaker.

3. Sprinkle a light layer on carpets where pet odor is an issue. Allow the blend to sit for 10 minutes to 1 hour, and then vacuum up. Repeat as needed.

# REFRIGERATOR CLEANSERS

Every so often, your refrigerator needs a good scrubbing, inside and out. In between deep cleanings, keep it looking and smelling fresh with these simple cleansers.

## Lemon-Basil Sanitizing Spray

Makes about 8 ounces

Perky lemon and fragrant basil sanitize your refrigerator inside and out, and leave it smelling fresh and clean.

7 ounces distilled water
1 ounce unflavored vodka
15 drops lemon essential oil
10 drops basil essential oil

1. In a bottle with a fine-mist spray top, combine all the ingredients. Shake well to blend, and then shake again before each use.

2. Apply 1 spritz to each area of your refrigerator you'd like to address. Wipe clean with a soft cloth or a paper towel. Repeat as needed.

## Quick Spot Cleaner

Makes 1 treatment

Sweet orange and baking soda make short work of sticky spills that happen around jelly jars, juice pitchers, and other containers.

1 tablespoon tap water
½ tablespoon baking soda
2 drops sweet orange essential oil

1. In a small dish, combine all the ingredients. Whisk to blend thoroughly.

2. With a soft scrub brush, apply the cleaner to the sticky spot, and allow it to sit for 30 seconds to 1 minute.

3. With the brush, vigorously scrub the affected area. Once all soil has loosened, use a cloth or paper towel soaked in warm tap water to wipe up. Repeat as needed.

## Minty Fresh Fridge

Makes 1 treatment

Spearmint and grapefruit combine with baking soda to absorb odors and leave your refrigerator smelling fresh and clean.

8 ounces baking soda
8 drops grapefruit essential oil
4 drops spearmint essential oil

1. In a medium bowl, combine all the ingredients. Whisk to blend thoroughly, and then transfer the mixture to a jar.

2. Place the uncovered jar in the back of the refrigerator where it will not be knocked over. Repeat once a month or as often as needed.

# RODENTS

No one wants to deal with dead mice, and poison pellets put your family, your pets, and wildlife at risk. Peppermint essential oil repels mice and rats better than any other natural option, keeping them out of your home. Here you have three different ways to use this powerful essential oil to suit your needs.

## Peppermint Mouse Bombs

Makes 8 reusable mouse bombs

Strong peppermint odors are too much for mice and rats to handle. One whiff, and they look for a different place to call home.

8 cotton balls
48 drops peppermint essential oil

1. On each cotton ball, place 6 drops of peppermint essential oil.

2. Place the mouse bombs in areas where you've seen signs of rodent activity.

3. Each evening, refresh the mouse bombs with 6 more drops of peppermint essential oil. You should see all activity cease within 3 to 4 days. Repeat as needed.

## Indoor/Outdoor Mouse Repellent

Makes 16 ounces

Diatomaceous earth holds scents in, and peppermint overpowers the sensitive noses of mice and rats. Spread this powder around potential entry points to keep rodents from welcoming themselves into your home.

2 cups diatomaceous earth
16 drops peppermint essential oil

1. In a medium bowl, combine all the ingredients. Stir well, and then transfer the powder to a glass or metal sugar shaker.

2. Apply a dusting of the repellent to outdoor areas where mice may be entering your home, especially around ducts, vents, and garage doors. Apply another dusting to indoor areas where you've seen signs of rodent activity. Leave the treatments in place until rodent activity stops. If it rains, reapply the outdoor treatment once the ground dries up. Repeat as needed.

## Mouse Repellent Spray

Makes about 8 ounces

Spray is a quick, easy way to apply peppermint essential oil to areas you can't quite reach, or where airflow makes other treatments impractical.

4 ounces distilled water
4 ounces rubbing alcohol
32 drops peppermint essential oil

1. In a bottle with a fine-mist spray top, combine all the ingredients. Shake well to blend, and then shake again before each use.

2. Apply 1 spritz to each area in your home where you've seen signs of rodent activity. Use a little more for large areas. Apply another spritz to each outdoor area where mice may be entering your home, especially around ducts, vents, and garage doors. Repeat as needed.

# SPIDERS

Spiders play an important role in nature's balance, but you probably don't want them inside your house. These simple repellents keep them away while helping keep your home smelling its best.

## Indoor Spider Repellent Spray

Makes about 8 ounces

Spiders hate peppermint and will go out of their way to avoid it. This spray is a quick, easy way to keep them out.

**4 ounces distilled water**
**4 ounces rubbing alcohol**
**25 drops peppermint essential oil**

1. In a bottle with a fine-mist spray top, combine all the ingredients. Shake well to blend, and then shake again before each use.

2. Apply 1 spritz to each area where spiders may be gaining access to your home, especially around ducts, vents, windows, and doors. Repeat as needed.

## Lemon-Mint Spider Repellent Powder

Makes 16 ounces

Peppermint and lemon deter spiders from making their way into your home. Spread this powder around the foundation to keep them out.

2 cups diatomaceous earth
16 drops peppermint essential oil
16 drops lemon essential oil

1. In a medium bowl, combine all the ingredients. Stir well, and then transfer the blend to a glass or metal sugar shaker.

2. Apply a dusting of repellent to the entire perimeter of your home. Pay special attention to areas near vents, windows, and doors. If it rains, reapply the outdoor treatment once the ground dries up. Repeat as needed.

## Synergistic Spider Spray

Makes about 8 ounces

Peppermint, eucalyptus, and tea tree essential oils combine to stop spiders in their tracks. This spray repels moths, silverfish, and cockroaches, too.

4 ounces distilled water
4 ounces rubbing alcohol
18 drops eucalyptus essential oil (any species)
12 drops peppermint essential oil
12 drops tea tree essential oil

1. In a bottle with a fine-mist spray top, combine all the ingredients. Shake well to blend, and then shake again before each use.

2. Apply 1 spritz to each area where spiders may be gaining access to your home, especially around ducts, vents, windows, and doors. Repeat as needed.

# STAIN REMOVERS

Despite our best efforts to stay tidy, life can be messy. Aromatherapy blends don't just smell good; many are ideal for removing tough stains.

## Bodily Fluids and Pet Accident Cleaner

Makes about 8 ounces

Lavender essential oil and white vinegar neutralize odors and remove urine and vomit stains quickly.

Baking soda (for stain coverage)
7 ounces white vinegar
1 ounce distilled water
20 drops lavender essential oil

1. Blot up any liquid with a paper towel, and discard it. Cover the area with a layer of baking soda and allow it to sit for 20 minutes.

2. In a bottle with a fine-mist spray top, combine all the ingredients. Shake well to blend, and then shake again before each use.

3. Use a paper towel to scoop up any liquid that the baking soda has absorbed and discard it. Apply 1 to 3 spritzes of the cleaner to the baking soda on top of the stain. Do not saturate the carpet with the vinegar solution. A light mist is all you need to get the mixture to bubble. When the bubbling action stops, wipe up the moisture and allow the area to dry.

4. Use a stiff brush to loosen remaining baking powder, and then vacuum. Repeat the treatment for deep stains. Use as often as needed.

## Lemon Grease Treatment

Makes 1 treatment

Lemon essential oil cuts through grease, making it easy to wash out. Even motor oil and black bicycle grease come out with lemon.

**1 drop lemon essential oil**

1. Apply the lemon essential oil straight from the bottle onto the grease spot. Use a little more for large spots.

2. On clothing, allow the essential oil to sit for 20 minutes, and then wash and dry the items as usual. On surfaces, allow the essential oil to sit for 20 minutes, and then use a soft scrub brush and some natural dish soap to break up the stain. Rinse the area with hot water when finished. Repeat as needed.

## Grass Stain Remover

Makes 1 treatment

Dirt, grass stains, and other organic materials, including fresh blood and red wine come right out with the help of lemon essential oil and a few laundry room basics.

**1 drop liquid castile soap**
**2 drops hydrogen peroxide**
**2 drops lemon essential oil**

1. In a small bottle, combine all the ingredients. Shake well to blend. Apply the remover to the grass-stained area, working it in with your fingers or a scrub brush.

2. Let the treatment sit for 3 minutes. With a scrub brush and cold water, scrub the stain from its outer edge in, and then rinse. Repeat as needed until the stain is gone.

# TOILETS

Commercial toilet cleaners do a good job of cleaning the commode, but aromatherapy solutions are better for you and for the planet. Thanks to their ability to kill bacteria, fungi, and viruses, you can stop spending money on chemical-laden cleaners.

## Lemon-Fresh Bleach Alternative

Makes about 6 cups

Besides leaving your toilet bowl sparkling clean, this lemon-fresh bleach alternative is safe for septic systems and laundry.

5 cups distilled water
4 ounces hydrogen peroxide
1 ounce lemon juice
5 drops lemon essential oil

1. In a bottle with a fine-mist spray top, combine all the ingredients. Shake well to blend, and then shake again before each use.
2. Spray the inside of the toilet bowl with the solution, and then use a toilet brush to scrub it clean. Repeat as needed.

## Hard Water Stain Scrub

Makes about 12 ounces

The natural acid in lemon essential oil cuts through grime, while Epsom salt and baking soda dissolve minerals and break up the hard water stains.

1 cup Epsom salt
½ cup baking soda
¼ cup liquid dish detergent
20 drops lemon essential oil

1. In a medium bowl, combine all the ingredients. Stir well, and then transfer the scrub to a plastic squeeze bottle.

2. Turn off the water source located behind the toilet, and then flush the toilet twice to leave the bare bowl exposed.

3. Apply 1 tablespoon of the mixture onto a damp scrub brush and apply it to the stain. Repeat until you have covered the entire toilet bowl.

4. Allow the mixture to sit for 10 to 15 minutes, and then use your brush to test a small area. If the stain starts to come off, scrub the whole toilet. If not, let the blend sit for another 10 to 15 minutes.

5. Scrub the entire toilet clean, and then turn the water source back on. After the tank fills, give the toilet a flush to rinse it. Repeat every few weeks to keep tough hard water stains at bay.

## Fresh Flush "No. 2" Spray

Makes 2 ounces

Elimination is completely natural, and so is the odor that usually accompanies it. However, if you spray this blend into the bowl before you go, no odor will escape. What's more, not only do bergamot, lemongrass, and grapefruit stop the odors, they also sanitize the toilet bowl.

1 tablespoon rubbing alcohol
6 drops grapefruit essential oil
2 drops bergamot essential oil
2 drops lemongrass essential oil
1 drop liquid castile soap
1½ ounces distilled water

1. In a bottle with a fine-mist spray top, combine the rubbing alcohol and the essential oils. Add the castile soap and the water, and swirl to blend.

2. Give the bottle a little shake before use, and then apply 1 or 2 spritzes to the water inside the toilet bowl before each bowel movement.

SUBSTITUTION TIP Any essential oil blend will work in this spray. Pick your favorites and substitute the oils drop for drop. A good combination to try is grapefruit, lemon, and mandarin; another is lavender, spearmint, and eucalyptus.

# UPHOLSTERY

Couch time is so much more pleasurable when there are no funky odors present. Skip the store-bought upholstery freshener, and allow aromatherapy blends to work their magic. You can even try these simple solutions in the car and on outdoor furniture cushions, too.

## Bergamot-Lime Upholstery Stain Remover

Makes about 10 ounces

Bergamot and lime give upholstery a fresh scent, while dish soap and borax help eliminate soil.

1 tablespoon borax
3 tablespoons liquid dish soap
1 cup boiling water
10 drops bergamot essential oil
5 drops lime essential oil

1. In a medium bowl, combine the borax and dish soap, and then add the boiling water. Whisk to blend thoroughly, ensuring that all the borax dissolves.

2. Wait for the blend to cool, and then transfer it to a bottle with a fine-mist spray top. Add the essential oils. Shake well to blend, and then shake again before each use.

3. Apply 1 to 3 spritzes onto a paper towel or cloth and wipe up spills on upholstery, working from the edge of the spill toward the center. Repeat as needed.

## Upholstery Freshening Spray

Makes 12 ounces

Commercial fabric freshening sprays often contain a surprisingly long list of toxic chemicals. This crisp citrus spray kills bacteria and deodorizes, leaving nothing but a clean smell behind.

1 cup distilled water
1 cup unflavored vodka
24 drops mandarin essential oil
12 drops grapefruit essential oil
4 drops lemon essential oil

1. In a bottle with a fine-mist spray top, combine all the ingredients. Shake well to blend, and then shake again before each use.

2. Lightly mist the item, ensuring that each area gets at least 1 spritz. Repeat as needed to keep upholstery smelling fresh.

PREFERENCE TIP Any combination of essential oils will work in this spray. Pick your favorites and substitute the oils suggested drop for drop. Enjoy.

## Lavender-Eucalyptus Upholstery Powder

Makes about 8 ounces

Musty smells can be difficult to remove with spray. Eucalyptus and lavender sanitize and leave a fresh fragrance behind, while baking powder absorbs tough odors.

1 cup baking soda
20 drops eucalyptus essential oil (any species)
10 drops lavender essential oil
1 teaspoon of uncooked rice
   (optional, for humidity control)

1. In a large bowl, combine all the ingredients. Whisk to blend thoroughly.

2. Sift the blend into a second bowl to eliminate lumps. If you are in a humid climate, add the rice to keep the powder from clumping, and mix in well. Transfer the mixture to a glass or metal sugar shaker.

3. Sprinkle a light layer onto upholstery, ensuring that you use enough to cover all areas. Work a little bit of powder down into the spaces between cushions.

4. Leave the powder in place for 1 hour, and then vacuum thoroughly. Repeat as needed.

# WOOD FURNITURE CARE

Instead of reaching for toxic commercial cleaners and polishes, mix up your own natural recipes. You'll love the way your wood furniture looks after one of these treatments, and you'll reap some aromatherapy benefits along the way.

## Vetiver-Myrrh Dusting Spray

Makes about 12 ounces

Not only do vetiver and myrrh smell amazing together, they also help you de-stress while you dust. When combined with simple kitchen ingredients, your dust-free furniture will glow.

1 cup distilled water
¼ cup white vinegar
2 tablespoons olive oil
15 drops myrrh essential oil
15 drops vetiver essential oil

1. In a bottle with a fine-mist spray top, combine all the ingredients. Shake well to blend, and then shake again before each use.

2. Spray a soft cloth with 1 to 3 spritzes of dusting spray and wipe surfaces clean. Repeat as needed.

## Tangerine-Bergamot Deep Cleaner

Makes about 4 ounces

Tangerine and bergamot promote feelings of elation, while a simple combination of olive oil and vinegar cleans grime off woodwork and furniture. Test this blend in a hidden area before using it on large areas.

¼ cup olive oil
¼ cup white vinegar
10 drops bergamot essential oil
10 drops tangerine essential oil

1. In a bottle with a narrow neck, combine all the ingredients. Shake well to blend, and then shake again before each use.

2. Apply ½ teaspoon of deep cleaner to a soft cloth, and scrub using circular motions. Repeat until the entire item is clean, and then use a soft cloth to buff off any remaining olive oil. Repeat as needed.

## Lemon Furniture Polish

Makes about 4 ounces

Lemon essential oil, beeswax, and coconut oil nourish wood and leave a deep, rich shine behind. Be sure to test this furniture polish on a hidden area before applying it to the entire piece.

2 ounces coconut oil, melted
1½ ounces beeswax, melted
½ ounce sweet almond oil
20 drops lemon essential oil

1. In a medium bowl, combine all the ingredients. Whisk to blend thoroughly, and then transfer the polish to a jar.

2. With a soft cloth, apply ½ teaspoon of the polish to the item. Use small, circular motions, applying more polish as needed. If your furniture is very thirsty, let the blend sit for 20 minutes before moving on to the next step.

3. When finished, buff the wood with a clean cloth to bring out the shine. Repeat as needed.

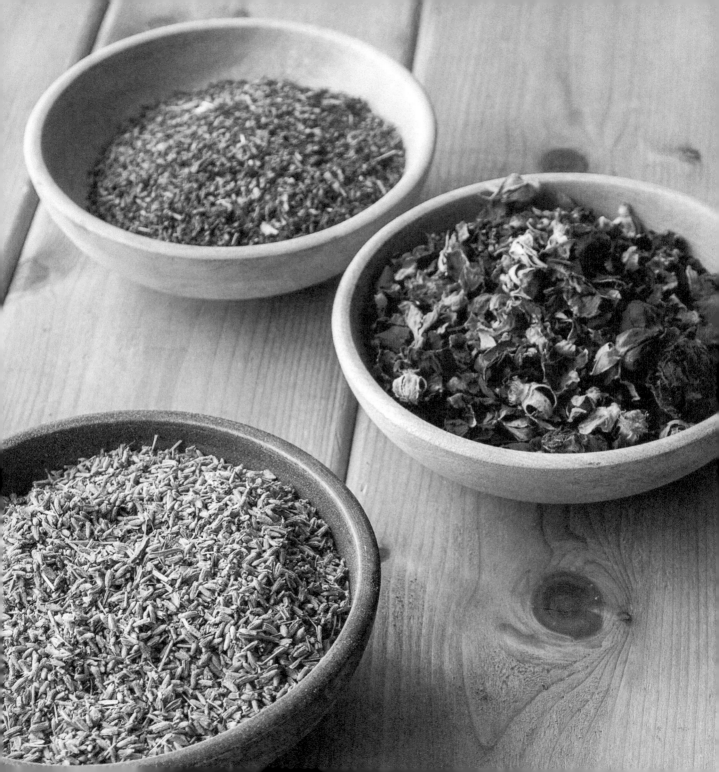

# SEVEN

# Essential Oil Profiles

Essential oils are the backbone of aromatherapy, and it's vital you learn the basics of each before using it on your skin or in your home. Each of the 85 short profiles found here covers important safety information and interesting facts about some of the most versatile and useful essential oils available, along with a list of medicinal properties, ideas for use, and inspiration for creating blends.

The botanical name is listed with each entry, along with a basic price estimate. Please note that prices can vary widely from one source to the next, and prices change along with market conditions.

$   *$15 and under*

$$   *$15–$30*

$$$   *$35–$50*

$$$$   *more than $50*

# ALLSPICE

*Pimenta dioica*

Spicy scent
Cost: $

Also known as pimenta or pimento berry, allspice essential oil is made from the leaves and/or fruit of an evergreen tree that grows primarily in South America and the West Indies. Its warm, pleasant fragrance helps with stress and mild depression, and is similar to the aroma of cloves. Allspice contains a high level of eugenol, which fights bacteria, numbs pain, and inhibits fungal growth, among other things. Eugenol is found in a variety of commercial products, including mouthwash and toothpaste.

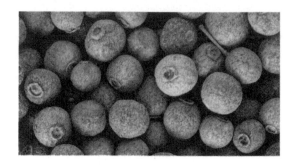

### MEDICINAL PROPERTIES
Analgesic, anesthetic, antiseptic, carminative, muscle relaxant, rubefacient, stimulant

### USES
Effective in treating bronchitis and sore muscles; ideal for making personal fragrances

### BLENDS WELL WITH
Bergamot, clove bud, geranium, ginger, jasmine, lavender, lemon, patchouli, sweet orange, ylang-ylang

### PRECAUTIONS
Do not use during pregnancy. Allspice can cause skin irritation if applied neat. Because it can irritate mucous membranes, it should not be inhaled directly.

# ANISE

*Pimpinella anisum*

Licorice scent
Cost: $

With a rich, sweet aroma reminiscent of authentic black licorice, anise has a long history in culinary and medicinal applications. Traditional liqueurs including arak, ouzo, pernod, and raki rely on the herb for their signature flavors. Anise is often sold as anise seed or aniseed essential oil. Be careful not to confuse it with star anise, or *Illicium verum*, because it offers different properties.

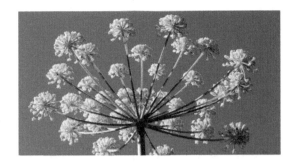

## MEDICINAL PROPERTIES
Antibacterial, antifungal, antiseptic, antispasmodic, aperient, aphrodisiac, carminative, cordial, decongestant, digestive, expectorant, insecticide, sedative, vermifuge

## USES
Effective in treating bronchitis, cold, and flu; ideal for treating ailments that include digestive discomfort

## BLENDS WELL WITH
Bay laurel, black pepper, fir needle, ginger, lavender, lime, pine, rose, spruce, sweet orange

## PRECAUTIONS
Do not use during pregnancy or if breastfeeding. Avoid if diagnosed with endometriosis or an estrogen-dependent form of cancer. Not recommended for children under 5 years old. Anise can irritate sensitive skin. Heavy doses have a narcotic effect, causing heartbeat and respiration to slow. Avoid if you are allergic to carrots, celery, or pollen. Use caution around pets; anise is toxic to birds and rodents.

# ATLAS CEDARWOOD

*Cedrus atlantica*

Woody scent
Cost: $

Atlas cedarwood has a long, storied history of use in architecture and furniture making, and these beautiful evergreen trees are popular with landscapers. Its woody, balsamic fragrance makes it a favorite in perfumery and incense making. Because both Atlas cedarwood and cedarwood essential oil from the *Cedrus deodara* species offer similar scents and medicinal properties, they are often interchangeable.

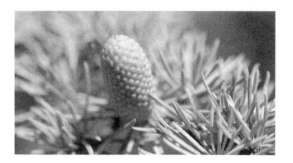

**MEDICINAL PROPERTIES**
Antibacterial, antifungal, anti-inflammatory, antiseptic, antispasmodic, aphrodisiac, astringent, diuretic, expectorant, insect repellent, insecticide, sedative, vulnerary

**USES**
Effective in treating acne, dandruff, and oily hair; ideal for making insect repellents

**BLENDS WELL WITH**
Bergamot, clary sage, cypress, frankincense, German chamomile, jasmine, juniper berry, lavender, neroli, palmarosa, petitgrain, Roman chamomile, rosemary, vetiver

**PRECAUTIONS**
Do not use during pregnancy. Atlas cedarwood can cause skin irritation if applied neat.

# BALSAM OF PERU

*Myroxylon balsamum*

Sweet vanilla scent

Cost: $

A wonderful essential oil for skin care, balsam of Peru also soothes feelings of minor depression, reduces stress, and promotes peaceful sleep. Its fragrance is strongly reminiscent of vanilla, with undertones of chocolate, making it a favorite with perfumeries and soap makers. It is considered an inexpensive substitute for costly vanilla essential oil.

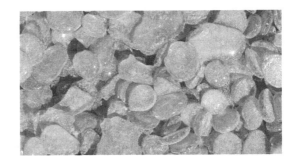

**MEDICINAL PROPERTIES**
Antibacterial, anti-inflammatory, antioxidant, antiseptic, cicatrizant, deodorant, diuretic, expectorant

**USES**
Effective in treating dry, chapped skin; ideal for making bath and body products

**BLENDS WELL WITH**
Atlas cedarwood, cardamom, cedarwood, cinnamon leaf, clove bud, ginger, lavender, lemon, lime, mandarin, marjoram, peppermint, rosemary, sweet orange, thyme

**PRECAUTIONS**
Balsam of Peru can cause skin sensitivity, especially in the elderly and children under 2 years old.

# BASIL

*Ocimum basilicum*

Sweet, herbaceous scent
Cost: $

Basil essential oil comes from the common culinary herb, which gets its name from the Greek word *basileum*, meaning king. A fantastic skin tonic for acne, it also relieves menstrual cramps, rheumatism, gout, and sore muscles. Basil should be avoided during pregnancy. However, when nursing, its use promotes greater milk production. In Italy, new moms traditionally eat basil leaves to stimulate lactation.

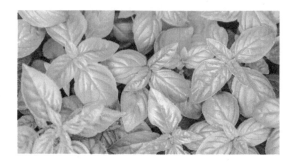

**MEDICINAL PROPERTIES**
Antibacterial, antidepressant, antiseptic, antispasmodic, digestive, expectorant, restorative, stomachic

**USES**
Effective in treating migraines, eliminating anxiousness, and soothing insect bites

**BLENDS WELL WITH**
Bay laurel, black pepper, citronella, lemon, lemongrass, lime, marjoram, melissa, oregano, peppermint, ravintsara, spearmint, vetiver, yuzu

**PRECAUTIONS**
Do not use during pregnancy.

# BAY LAUREL

*Laurus nobilis*

Spicy, sweet scent
Cost: $

Also known as sweet bay or laurel leaf, bay laurel essential oil offers an uplifting fragrance, with hints of camphor and spice. Sourced from the same plant as bay leaves used for culinary purposes, this essential oil is ideal for diffusing when you have a cold or the flu. You can also diffuse it when you're feeling stressed and on the edge of illness; it supports a healthy immune system while promoting clarity and peace of mind.

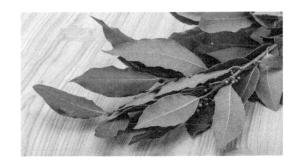

## MEDICINAL PROPERTIES
Analgesic, antibacterial, antiseptic, antispasmodic, antiviral, astringent, cholagogue, emmenagogue, expectorant, febrifuge, insecticide, sedative, stomachic, sudorific

## USES
Effective in treating cold and flu; ideal for supporting digestive health

## BLENDS WELL WITH
Bergamot, clary sage, cypress, eucalyptus, frankincense, ginger, juniper berry, lavender, lemon, myrtle, patchouli, pine, ravensara leaf, ravintsara, rosemary, Spanish sage, sweet orange, ylang-ylang

## PRECAUTIONS
Do not use during pregnancy. Bay laurel can cause skin irritation.

# BENZOIN

*Styrax benzoin, S. tonkinensis*

Warm, sweet scent
Cost: $$

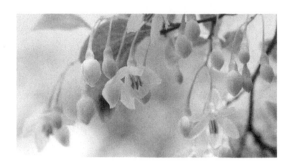

With a pleasant aroma that carries a strong hint of vanilla, benzoin essential oil is very popular with perfumeries and incense makers. Historically used in India and Asia, it was also quite popular with ancient Egyptians. It is no surprise, then, that this beautiful oil is ideal for alleviating stress and creating a sense of euphoria.

### MEDICINAL PROPERTIES
Antidepressant, anti-inflammatory, antiseptic, astringent, carminative, cordial, deodorant, diuretic, expectorant, sedative, vulnerary

### USES
Effective in treating arthritis, rheumatism, body aches, and joint pains; ideal for relieving chapped, dry skin

### BLENDS WELL WITH
Bergamot, black pepper, cinnamon leaf, coriander, cypress, frankincense, ginger, jasmine, juniper berry, lavender, lemon, marjoram, myrrh, petitgrain, rose, rosemary, sandalwood, sweet orange

### PRECAUTIONS
Avoid use before driving or undertaking important tasks.

# BERGAMOT

*Citrus bergamia*

Spicy, citrus scent
Cost: $$

A valuable essential oil for treating oily skin, abscesses, and boils, bergamot is also a good choice for dealing with stress and exhaustion. If you suffer from seasonal depression, you may find that diffusing bergamot is a good way to lift your mood and give you the inspiration you need to get up and go. Choose bergamot FCF, which stands for furocoumarin free, if possible; it has had the bergaptene (furocoumarin) removed, and is far less phototoxic than standard bergamot.

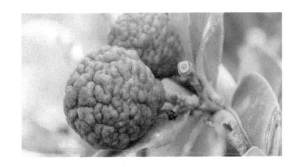

### MEDICINAL PROPERTIES
Analgesic, antidepressant, antiseptic, antispasmodic, calmative, cicatrizant, deodorant, digestive, febrifuge, stomachic, vermifuge, vulnerary

### USES
Effective in treating acne, oily skin, psoriasis, and eczema; ideal for making bath and body products

### BLENDS WELL WITH
Basil, clary sage, coriander, cypress, geranium, German chamomile, ginger, hops flower, jasmine, juniper berry, palo santo, Roman chamomile, rose, sandalwood, vetiver

### PRECAUTIONS
Phototoxic if not labeled "bergamot FCF"; do not apply to skin that will be exposed to direct sunlight. Bergamot can cause sensitive skin.

# BLACK PEPPER

*Piper nigrum*

Warm, spicy scent
Cost: $

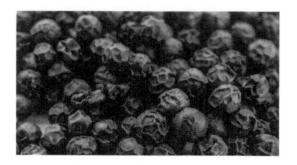

Offering a crisp, spicy scent with hints of green and the slightest touch of flowers, black pepper essential oil smells a little bit like freshly ground peppercorns. It stimulates the mind and promotes alertness. Its ability to facilitate circulation while providing a deep, warming effect makes it a good choice in blends designed to ease muscle pain and aching joints.

### MEDICINAL PROPERTIES
Analgesic, antiseptic, antispasmodic, aphrodisiac, diaphoretic, digestive, diuretic, febrifuge, laxative, rubefacient

### USES
Effective in treating digestive problems, arthritis, flu, and cold; ideal for use in blends designed to provide emotional motivation

### BLENDS WELL WITH
Bergamot, clary sage, clove bud, coriander, fennel seed, frankincense, geranium, ginger, grapefruit, juniper berry, lavender, lemon, lime, mandarin, sandalwood, Spanish sage, rosewood, ylang-ylang

### PRECAUTIONS
Avoid topical use during pregnancy due to increased risk of skin sensitization. Black pepper can cause sensitive skin.

# CAJUPUT

*Melaleuca leucadendron, M. minor*

Sweet, camphorous scent
Cost: $

Also known as cajeput, or *Melaleuca minor,* cajuput essential oil relieves cold and flu symptoms including congestion and sore throat. A close relative to tea tree, it is also suitable for treating asthma and bronchitis, muscle aches, and oily skin. Its sweet, lightly camphorous aroma promotes a clear, alert state of mind, and makes it an excellent choice for use in natural insect repellents.

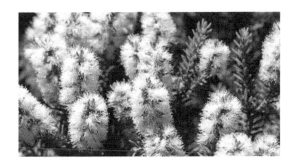

**MEDICINAL PROPERTIES**
Analgesic, antiseptic, antispasmodic, carminative, decongestant, expectorant, febrifuge, insect repellent, insecticide, stimulant, sudorific, vermifuge

**USES**
Effective in treating skin conditions such as acne, eczema, and psoriasis; ideal for making insect repellents

**BLENDS WELL WITH**
Bergamot, citronella, clary sage, clove bud, geranium, lavender, lemongrass, rosemary, thyme, vetiver

**PRECAUTIONS**
Avoid topical use during pregnancy due to increased risk of skin sensitization. Cajuput can cause skin irritation when used at high concentrations.

# CARAWAY SEED

*Carum carvi*

Sweet, spicy scent
Cost: $

A wonderfully energizing essential oil, caraway seed offers an aroma that has variously been described as spicy and sweet, fruity, peppery, and herbaceous. It makes an intriguing addition to personal scents and when diffused, it proves useful in easing laryngitis, bronchitis, and cold symptoms.

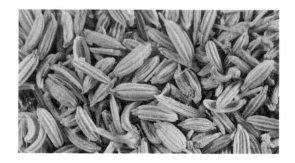

### MEDICINAL PROPERTIES
Antihistaminic, antiseptic, antispasmodic, aperitif, astringent, carminative, digestive, disinfectant, diuretic, emmenagogue, expectorant, galactagogue, stimulant, stomachic, vermifuge

### USES
Effective in treating digestive ailments and gastric spasms; ideal for soothing mental fatigue

### BLENDS WELL WITH
Basil, coriander, frankincense, German chamomile, ginger, lavender, Roman chamomile, sweet orange

### PRECAUTIONS
Do not use during pregnancy. Caraway seed can cause skin irritation when used at high concentrations.

# CARDAMOM
*Elettaria cardamomum*

Sweet, spicy scent
Cost: $$

You might recognize cardamom as one of the spices that gives chai tea its irresistible flavor. Cardamom essential oil comes from the seeds of a perennial herb with a reed-like structure. Highly prized by Egyptians for perfumery and incense, these seeds were also chewed as tooth whiteners, and Romans nibbled on them to ease indigestion.

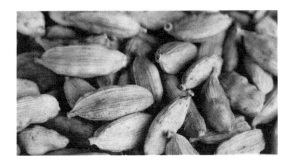

MEDICINAL PROPERTIES
Antiseptic, antispasmodic, carminative, cephalic, digestive, diuretic, expectorant, stimulant, stomachic

USES
Effective in treating nausea and indigestion; ideal for making refreshing bath and body products

BLENDS WELL WITH
Bergamot, caraway seed, cedarwood, cinnamon leaf, clove bud, hops flower, lime, mandarin, rose, spikenard, sweet orange, tangerine

PRECAUTIONS
Generally regarded as safe.

# CARROT SEED

*Daucus carota*

Earthy, herbaceous scent
Cost: $$

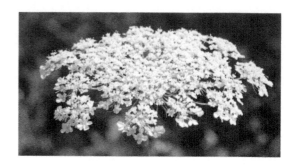

Primarily obtained from European wild carrots, carrot seed essential oil is sometimes confused with inexpensive carrot oil, which is a macerated infusion of domestic carrots and carrier oil. Carrot seed essential oil contains high levels of carotene and vitamin A. Its ability to stimulate and rejuvenate skin makes it a valuable addition to bath and body products, and combining it with complementary essential oils such as geranium and rose is an excellent tactic for naturally reducing the appearance of wrinkles.

## MEDICINAL PROPERTIES
Antiseptic, carminative, cytophylactic, depurative, diuretic, emmenagogue, hepatic, stimulant, vermifuge

## USES
Effective in treating dermatitis, rashes, and eczema; ideal for making rejuvenating bath and body products

## BLENDS WELL WITH
Atlas cedarwood, bergamot, caraway seed, cardamom, cedarwood, cinnamon leaf, clove bud, geranium, ginger, juniper berry, lavender, lemon, lime, mandarin, rose, rose geranium, sweet orange

## PRECAUTIONS
Do not use during pregnancy.

# CATNIP

*Nepeta cataria*

Minty, herbaceous scent
Cost: $$

Sometimes referred to as catmint,
catnip is highly stimulating to felines,
but sometimes has the opposite effect
on humans, promoting feelings of
relaxed well-being. Some migraine
sufferers find that applying a drop
or two of diluted catnip essential oil
stops their pain quickly.

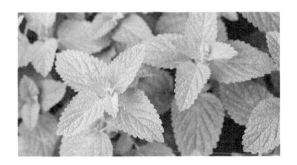

MEDICINAL PROPERTIES
Anesthetic, anti-inflammatory, antispasmodic,
astringent, carminative, emmenagogue,
nervine, sedative

USES
Effective in treating headaches, cramps, and
minor sprains; ideal for making natural insect
repellent

BLENDS WELL WITH
Eucalyptus, grapefruit, lavender, lemon,
lime, marjoram, myrrh, peppermint, rosemary,
spearmint, sweet orange

PRECAUTIONS
Do not use during pregnancy. Catnip can cause
skin irritation. This oil must be heavily diluted
before being used around cats.

# CEDARWOOD

*Juniperus virginiana*

Soft, woody scent
Cost: $

Sometimes confused with Atlas cedarwood, this essential oil comes from Virginian red cedar trees, which are also known as eastern red, Bedford, or southern red cedars. Prized by Native Americans, the oldest examples of these trees are estimated to have sprouted over 900 years ago. Like many other products made with this beautiful red wood, cedarwood essential oil deters insect activity. Meanwhile, its soft fragrance helps soothe nervous tension and ease anxiety.

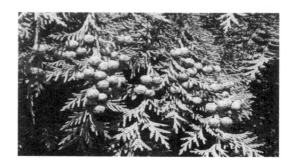

### MEDICINAL PROPERTIES
Antiseborrheic, antiseptic, antispasmodic, astringent, diuretic, emmenagogue, expectorant, fungicide, insect repellent, insecticide, sedative

### USES
Effective in treating arthritis, respiratory illnesses, and UTIs; ideal for making products to combat oily skin and hair

### BLENDS WELL WITH
Benzoin, bergamot, cinnamon leaf, citronella, cypress, frankincense, helichrysum, jasmine, juniper berry, lavender, lemon, lime, neroli, rose, rose geranium, rosemary

### PRECAUTIONS
Do not use during pregnancy. Cedarwood can cause skin irritation when used at high concentrations.

# CINNAMON LEAF

*Cinnamomum zeylanicum, C. verum*

Warm, spicy scent
Cost: $

While cinnamon leaf essential oil comes from the same trees as cinnamon bark oil does, it has a higher eugenol content that increases its value as a topical analgesic. As a spice, cinnamon finds its way into sweet and savory dishes that span cultures worldwide. The essential oil was historically used for a variety of purposes, ranging from temple incense to massaging sore feet.

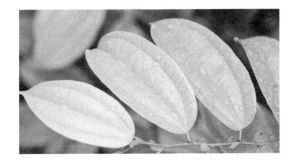

## MEDICINAL PROPERTIES
Analgesic, antibiotic, antiseptic, antispasmodic, aphrodisiac, astringent, carminative, emmenagogue, insecticide, stimulant, stomachic, vermifuge

## USES
Effective in treating joint and muscle pain, cramps, and painful periods; ideal In aromatherapy blends for respiratory ailments and depression

## BLENDS WELL WITH
Balsam of Peru, benzoin, cardamom, clove bud, coriander, frankincense, ginger, grapefruit, lavender, lemon, mandarin, petitgrain, rosemary, sweet orange, tangerine, thyme, ylang-ylang

## PRECAUTIONS
Do not use during pregnancy. Cinnamon leaf can cause severe skin irritation and mucous membrane irritation when used at high concentrations.

# CITRONELLA

*Cymbopogon nardus,*
*Andropogon nardus*

Sweet, citrus scent
Cost: $

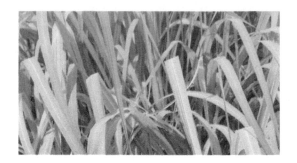

Citronella essential oil comes from a fragrant, tropical grass that has been employed in culinary and medicinal roles for thousands of years. Popular throughout China, Africa, and Southeast Asia, it is used for a wide range of ailments that includes fevers, headaches, and menstrual problems, along with digestive illnesses. In the Western world, its greatest value lies in its efficacy as an insect repellent.

MEDICINAL PROPERTIES
Antiseptic, antiviral, bactericidal, deodorant, diaphoretic, febrifuge, insect repellent, insecticide, stimulant

USES
Effective in treating cold, fever, and flu; ideal for use in refreshing bath and body products that double as insect repellents

BLENDS WELL WITH
Atlas cedarwood, bergamot, cedarwood, cypress, fir needle, frankincense, geranium, lavender, lemon, lemon eucalyptus, lemongrass, pine, sandalwood, vetiver

PRECAUTIONS
Citronella can cause sensitive skin.

# CLARY SAGE

*Salvia sclarea*

Herbaceous, slightly fruity scent
Cost: $$

Clary sage is an excellent essential oil for relaxation, and when used in bedtime blends, it can lull you gently to sleep. It is most popular, though, for its value in treating PMS, painful periods, and menopause symptoms. It contains sclareol, a constituent with an estrogen-like structure that helps bring hormones into balance. When diffused or worn in personal fragrance blends, clary sage can promote a calm feeling of self-confidence.

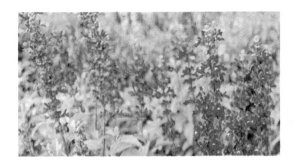

### MEDICINAL PROPERTIES
Antidepressant, anti-inflammatory, antiseptic, antispasmodic, aphrodisiac, astringent, bactericidal, carminative, deodorant, digestive, emmenagogue, euphoric, hypotensive, nervine, parturient, sedative, stomachic

### USES
Effective in treating depression and postnatal depression; ideal for making relaxing bath and body products

### BLENDS WELL WITH
Bergamot, cedarwood, frankincense, geranium, juniper berry, lavender, lemon, sandalwood, sweet orange, vitex berry

### PRECAUTIONS
Do not use during pregnancy. Do not use before driving or operating machinery.

# CLOVE BUD

*Eugenia caryophyllata, Syzygium aromaticum*

Sweet, spicy scent
Cost: $

The irresistible aroma of clove bud essential oil stimulates the mind and helps lift depression; however, its greatest value lies in its ability to aid digestion and ease physical discomfort. An excellent remedy for dental pain, it is also ideal for soothing stiff, aching muscles and joints. Placed on a cotton ball, a few drops of clove bud essential oil will fragrance a linen cabinet while keeping insects away.

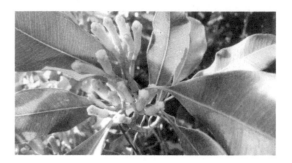

### MEDICINAL PROPERTIES
Analgesic, antifungal, antiseptic, antispasmodic, carminative, disinfectant, insecticide, stimulant, stomachic

### USES
Effective in treating athlete's foot, toothache, and digestive complaints; ideal for making warming massage blends to ease muscle pain, cramping, and spasms

### BLENDS WELL WITH
Allspice, basil, benzoin, bergamot, cinnamon leaf, clary sage, ginger, helichrysum, hops flower, lavender, lemon, lime, myrtle, sandalwood, sweet orange, yuzu

### PRECAUTIONS
Do not use during pregnancy. Do not use if diagnosed with liver or kidney disease. Clove bud can cause skin irritation and mucous membrane irritation when used at high concentrations.

# COPAIBA

*Copaifera reticulata*

Mild, woody scent
Cost: $–$$$

Traditionally used by Brazilian natives to heal skin, copaiba has a very mild, almost wet-smelling wood aroma that blends very well with almost all other fragrances. It's advisable to use a little at a time because the scent gets stronger when exposed to air or placed on skin.

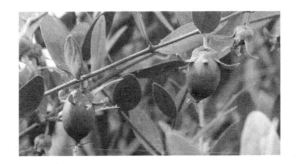

**MEDICINAL PROPERTIES**
Antibacterial, anti-inflammatory, decongestant, disinfectant, diuretic, expectorant, stimulant

**USES**
Effective in treating intestinal issues, including diarrhea; ideal for making anti-anxiety blends and blends to increase concentration while alleviating stress

**BLENDS WELL WITH**
Atlas cedarwood, bay laurel, bergamot, carrot seed, cedarwood, cinnamon leaf, clary sage, frankincense, lavender, mandarin, palmarosa

**PRECAUTIONS**
Do not use during pregnancy. Undiluted copaiba can cause sensitive skin.

# CORIANDER

*Coriandrum sativum*

Sweet, spicy scent
Cost: $$

If coriander's name sounds familiar to you, it's probably because of its use as a culinary spice. Ancient Greeks and Romans used coriander to give wine's flavor more depth, and it is a flavoring component in Benedictine and Chartreuse liqueurs. Beyond its use as a flavoring agent, coriander eases indigestion, diarrhea, and nausea, and its warming action has a therapeutic effect on muscle pain.

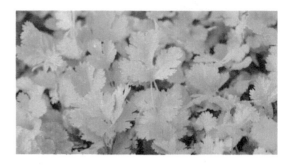

### MEDICINAL PROPERTIES
Analgesic, antispasmodic, aphrodisiac, carminative, deodorant, depurative, digestive, fungicidal, stimulant, stomachic

### USES
Effective in treating coughs, headaches, and mental fatigue; ideal for making warming massage blends

### BLENDS WELL WITH
Bergamot, cajuput, cinnamon leaf, eucalyptus (all types), ginger, grapefruit, lavender, lemon, lemongrass, lime, May Chang, neroli, sandalwood, spikenard, sweet orange

### PRECAUTIONS
Generally regarded as safe.

# CUCUMBER SEED

*Cucumis sativus*

Sweet, refreshing scent

Cost: $

Cucumbers are enjoyed worldwide for their refreshing flavor, and they have a long history of use in facemasks and rejuvenating skin treatments. Cucumber seed essential oil has a bright, uplifting fragrance and, thanks to its high level of vitamin C and omega-6 fatty acid, it makes a marvelous addition to cleansers, facial toners, and moisturizers.

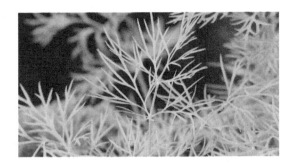

## MEDICINAL PROPERTIES
Anti-inflammatory, antioxidant, antiseptic, diuretic

## USES
Effective in treating psoriasis, acne, sunburn, and stretch marks; ideal for making nourishing hair and body products

## BLENDS WELL WITH
Bergamot, carrot seed, geranium, grapefruit, lavender, lemon, lime, mandarin, neroli, sweet orange, ylang-ylang

## PRECAUTIONS
Generally regarded as safe.

# CYPRESS

*Cupressus sempervirens*

Woody, slightly spicy scent
Cost: $

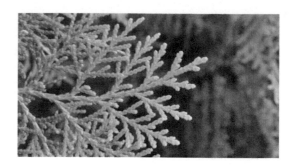

Besides offering a very versatile essential oil, cypress has a fascinating history. Thanks to the wood's durability and resilience, it was used to carve Egyptian sarcophagi, and ancient Greeks often used it to carve statues of their gods. Because of its association with cemeteries and grave goods, cypress is nicknamed the "tree of death," but its botanical name alludes to its long life. Cypress essential oil has a long litany of uses, benefiting ailments as varied as hemorrhoids, muscle cramps, and stress.

## MEDICINAL PROPERTIES
Antiseptic, antispasmodic, astringent, calmative, deodorant, diuretic, hemostatic, hepatic, insect repellent, insecticide, sedative, styptic, sudorific, vasoconstrictor

## USES
Effective in treating varicose veins, asthma, bronchitis, and flu; ideal for making massage blends for muscle aches and cramping

## BLENDS WELL WITH
Bergamot, clary sage, copaiba, frankincense, helichrysum, juniper berry, lavender, marjoram, myrtle, pine, ravensara leaf, rosemary, sandalwood, sweet orange, yuzu

## PRECAUTIONS
Avoid topical use during pregnancy due to increased risk of skin sensitization. Cypress essential oil gets stronger with age, so the older the oil, the less you'll need.

# DAVANA

*Artemisia pallens*

Green, herbal scent
Cost: $$$

While davana is expensive, it makes a fascinating addition to bath and body blends, as its aroma smells different on every wearer. If you are interested in making your own perfumes, then davana should be on your list of must-haves. Beyond its usefulness in perfumery, davana essential oil is a strong antidepressant, and its antiviral and antiseptic properties make it useful in treating a variety of illnesses.

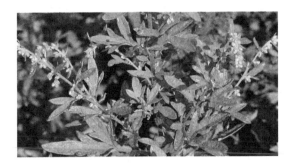

### MEDICINAL PROPERTIES
Antiviral, disinfectant, emmenagogue, expectorant, relaxant, vulnerary

### USES
Effective in treating minor wounds, muscle cramps, and headaches; ideal for making delightful personalized perfumes

### BLENDS WELL WITH
Allspice, Atlas cedarwood, bergamot, cedarwood, cypress, geranium, grapefruit, mandarin, neroli, palo santo, rose, rose geranium, rosewood, sweet orange, tangerine, ylang-ylang, yuzu

### PRECAUTIONS
Do not use during pregnancy. Davana can cause sensitive skin.

# DILL SEED

*Anethum graveolens*

Fresh, herbaceous scent
Cost: $$

While dill seed is commonly put to culinary use and its aroma might automatically remind you of home-made pickles, its usefulness extends far beyond the kitchen. It is an effective treatment for nausea and indigestion, and is gentle enough for use on young children. If you're trying to lose weight, you'll appreciate its ability to curb your appetite and help ease water retention.

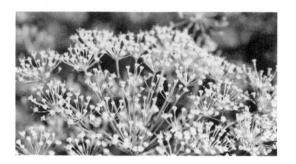

MEDICINAL PROPERTIES
Antibacterial, antioxidant, antiseptic, anti-spasmodic, aperitif, carminative, digestive, disinfectant, diuretic, emmenagogue, galactagogue, laxative, sedative, stomachic

USES
Effective in treating a wide range of digestive complaints

BLENDS WELL WITH
Bergamot, caraway, coriander, lemon, lime

PRECAUTIONS
Do not use during pregnancy. Dill seed can be very relaxing and may slow your reflexes; be mindful of how it affects you before driving or operating machinery.

# ELEMI

*Canarium luzonicum*

Fresh, citrus-like scent
Cost: $

The elemi tree is in the same family as frankincense and myrrh. Not only did ancient Egyptians use it in embalming, but they valued it for its usefulness in skin care, medicinal salves, incense, and more. In the Middle East, elemi was used as an antiseptic and healing agent. Today, it remains an excellent choice for skincare, and it makes a valuable addition to your cold and flu arsenal.

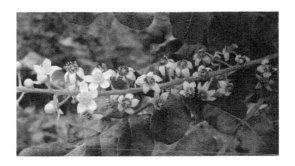

### MEDICINAL PROPERTIES
Analgesic, antiseptic, expectorant, stimulant

### USES
Effective in treating respiratory ailments, excess mucus, and minor wounds; ideal for making rejuvenating bath and body products

### BLENDS WELL WITH
Cardamom, carrot seed, cinnamon leaf, clary sage, clove bud, cucumber seed, frankincense, geranium, helichrysum, lavender, myrrh, rose, rose geranium, rosemary, Spanish sage

### PRECAUTIONS
Elemi can cause sensitive skin.

# EUCALYPTUS GLOBULUS

*Eucalyptus globulus*

Crisp, camphorous scent
Cost: $

Of the many types of eucalyptus essential oil commonly offered for sale, *Eucalyptus globulus* is among the most popular. It offers a variety of medicinal actions, and its ability to reduce swelling of the mucous membranes makes it a valuable ally during cold and flu season. Topically, it eases inflammation and muscle soreness.

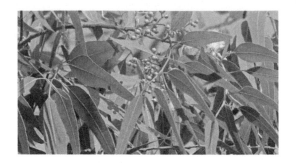

### MEDICINAL PROPERTIES
Analgesic, antibacterial, anti-inflammatory, antiseptic, antispasmodic, antiviral, astringent, cicatrizant, decongestant, deodorant, depurative, diuretic, expectorant, febrifuge, rubefacient, stimulant, vermifuge, vulnerary

### USES
Effective in treating headaches, asthma, sinusitis, and congestion; ideal for making healing salves for burns, blisters, insect bites, and minor wounds

### BLENDS WELL WITH
Benzoin, cajuput, lavender, lemongrass, lemon, pine, rosemary, tea tree, thyme

### PRECAUTIONS
Do not use on children under six years old. Avoid if diagnosed with epilepsy or high blood pressure. Excessive use of eucalyptus can cause headaches.

# EUCALYPTUS RADIATA

*Eucalyptus radiata*

Soft, camphorous scent
Cost: $

Offering a softer fragrance than its close cousin, *Eucalyptus globulus, Eucalyptus radiata* is a milder choice for treating upper respiratory issues, particularly in children and the elderly. Diffuse or vaporize it to clear a stuffy nose, or blend it into a soothing massage oil to ease the pain of arthritis or rheumatism.

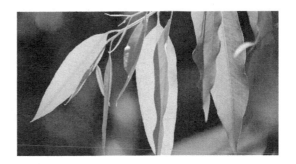

### MEDICINAL PROPERTIES
Antibacterial, antifungal, anti-inflammatory, antiviral, insect repellent, stimulant

### USES
Effective in treating minor cuts and scrapes; ideal for diffusing during cold and flu season

### BLENDS WELL WITH
Bergamot, black pepper, cajuput, German chamomile, ginger, marjoram, peppermint, pine, Roman chamomile, spearmint, spruce

### PRECAUTIONS
Do not use on children less than three years old. Avoid if diagnosed with diabetes, as it can raise blood sugar in diabetics. Asthmatics sometimes react to *Eucalyptus radiata*; proceed with caution if you have asthma.

# FENNEL SEED

*Foeniculum vulgare*

Sweet, peppery scent
Cost: $

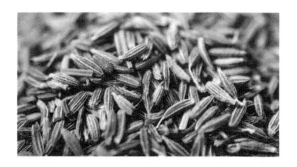

Also known as sweet fennel, this intriguing essential oil is excellent for addressing digestive issues. Besides helping with nausea, vomiting, flatulence, and hiccups, fennel seed can help with appetite control. Roman soldiers ate the seeds to keep hunger pangs at bay while on long marches, and early Christians chewed fennel seed to stave off hunger during periods of fasting.

### MEDICINAL PROPERTIES
Antiseptic, antispasmodic, carminative, depurative, diuretic, emmenagogue, expectorant, galactagogue, laxative, stimulant, stomachic, vermifuge

### USES
Effective in treating bloating, constipation, and indigestion; ideal for making skincare products to sort out oily skin, fight wrinkles, and smooth cellulite

### BLENDS WELL WITH
Bergamot, black pepper, cardamom, cypress, dill seed, fir needle, geranium, ginger, grapefruit, hops flower, juniper berry, lavender, lemon, mandarin, marjoram, niaouli, orange, pine, ravensara leaf, rose, rose geranium, rosemary, tangerine, ylang-ylang

### PRECAUTIONS
Do not use during pregnancy. Avoid if diagnosed with epilepsy or an estrogen-dependent form of cancer.

# FIR NEEDLE

*Abies balsamea*

Fresh conifer scent
Cost: $

Also known as European silver fir,
white spruce, or white fir, the tree
that produces this fragrant essential
oil was historically used for a variety of health purposes. Its buds and
bark were used in antiseptics, and its
resin, bark, and needles were used
for conditions ranging from muscle
pain to fever. Like the tree, fir needle
essential oil offers a variety of aromatherapy benefits, and its beautiful,
green, forest fragrance makes it a
pleasure to use.

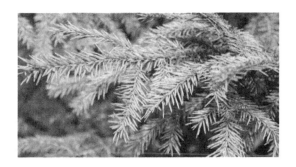

**MEDICINAL PROPERTIES**
Analgesic, antiseptic, astringent, decongestant,
deodorant, diuretic, expectorant, rubefacient,
stimulant, vasoconstrictor, vulnerary

**USES**
Effective in treating upper respiratory illnesses;
ideal for making balms, salves, and compresses
for pain relief

**BLENDS WELL WITH**
Atlas cedarwood, benzoin, cedarwood, copaiba,
cypress, davana, juniper berry, lavender, lemon,
marjoram, oregano, peppermint, pine, rosemary, spearmint, spruce, sweet orange

**PRECAUTIONS**
Fir needle can cause sensitive skin.

# FRANKINCENSE

*Boswellia carterii*

Spicy, woody scent
Cost: $$

Frankincense has been used in incense for thousands of years, and it is also used to treat a variety of skin ailments. Its ability to calm the mind and create inner peace makes it a valuable oil to diffuse during meditation and its mild sedative property encourages deep, slow breathing. Combined with its expectorant and antiseptic properties, this makes it ideal for treating respiratory illnesses.

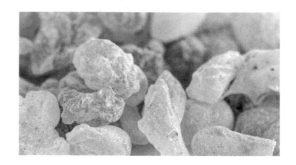

### MEDICINAL PROPERTIES
Antiseptic, astringent, carminative, cicatrizant, cytophylactic, digestive, diuretic, emmenagogue, expectorant, sedative, vulnerary

### USES
Effective in treating asthma, bronchitis, cough, cold, and laryngitis; ideal for making healing balms and salves for wounds, scars, aging skin, and inflammation

### BLENDS WELL WITH
Bergamot, black pepper, cinnamon leaf, cypress, geranium, grapefruit, helichrysum, lavender, lemon, mandarin, neroli, orange, palmarosa, patchouli, pine, rose, rose geranium, sandalwood, vetiver, ylang-ylang

### PRECAUTIONS
Do not use during pregnancy.

# GALBANUM

*Ferula galbaniflua*

Green, woody scent
Cost: $$

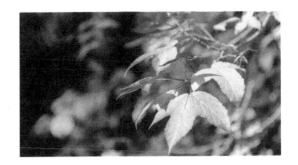

Ancient Romans and Greeks burned galbanum resin as incense, mixed the fragrant oil into their baths, and used it to formulate healing balms and decadent perfumes. Galbanum essential oil is a wonderful tonic for weary minds, and as it stimulates circulation, eases inflammation, and helps wounds heal faster while diminishing the appearance of scars.

## MEDICINAL PROPERTIES
Antispasmodic, cicatrizant, decongestant, detoxifier, emollient, insect repellent, insecticide, vermifuge, vulnerary

## USES
Effective in treating arthritis, rheumatism, and gout; ideal for diffusion and vapor treatments for treating upper respiratory issues

## BLENDS WELL WITH
Allspice, benzoin, cardamom, elemi, fir needle, frankincense, geranium, ginger, lavender, palmarosa, palo santo, pine, rose geranium, sweet orange

## PRECAUTIONS
Generally regarded as safe.

# GERANIUM

*Pelargonium odoratissimum*

Fresh, faintly floral scent
Cost: $

Offering an irresistible, intriguing fragrance, geranium is a versatile essential oil useful for making insect repellent, creating comforting skincare products to deal with dry or aging skin, and distilling for clean, fresh-smelling indoor air. This beautiful oil also offers relief from physical discomfort; its hormone-balancing qualities make it a good choice for treating PMS, painful periods, breast engorgement, and menopause symptoms.

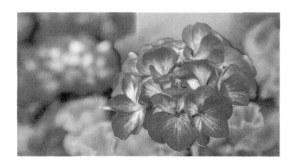

## MEDICINAL PROPERTIES
Antiseptic, astringent, cicatrizant, cytophylactic, deodorant, diuretic, hemostatic, styptic, tonic, vermifuge, vulnerary

## USES
Effective in treating eczema and shingles; ideal for easing stress, anxiety, and tension

## BLENDS WELL WITH
Atlas cedarwood, bergamot, carrot seed, cedarwood, clary sage, cucumber seed, grapefruit, helichrysum, jasmine, juniper berry, lavender, lime, melissa, neroli, petitgrain, ravensara leaf, rose, rosemary, sandalwood, sweet orange

## PRECAUTIONS
Not recommended for use during pregnancy due to geranium's hormone-balancing effect. Not recommended if diagnosed with diabetes, as geranium can reduce blood sugar.

# GERMAN CHAMOMILE

*Matricaria recutita*

Strong, sweet, herbaceous scent
Cost: $$$

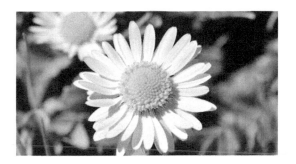

If you have ever spent time relaxing with a cup of hot chamomile tea, you have probably felt the wonderfully relaxing quality of German chamomile at work. Besides offering gentle sedation, particularly at bedtime or when suffering from a nasty cold, German chamomile contains levomenol, which helps heal compromised skin. Also known as blue chamomile, German chamomile essential oil gets its vivid color from azulene, which imparts a potent anti-inflammatory effect.

**MEDICINAL PROPERTIES**
Analgesic, anti-allergenic, antibiotic, anti-inflammatory, antispasmodic, bactericidal, carminative, cholagogue, cicatrizant, digestive, emmenagogue, hepatic, sedative, stomachic, vasoconstrictor, vermifuge, vulnerary

**USES**
Effective in treating inflamed skin, psoriasis, and eczema

**BLENDS WELL WITH**
Benzoin, bergamot, clary sage, frankincense, geranium, grapefruit, helichrysum, jasmine, lavender, lemon, lime, mandarin, marjoram, neroli, patchouli, ravintsara, rose, rosemary, sweet orange, tea tree, ylang-ylang

**PRECAUTIONS**
Do not use during pregnancy.

# GINGER

*Zingiber officinale*

Warm, spicy scent
Cost: $

Ginger is a tropical perennial herb that bears fragrant flowers and a crown of narrow, spear-shaped leaves. While it is prized for its aboveground beauty and aroma, the spice and essential oil comes from its roots, which are thick, spreading rhizomes. Ginger has been used medicinally for millennia, with mentions in Chinese and Sanskrit texts as well as in ancient Roman, Greek, and Arabian literature. The plant's name is derived from India's Gingee district, where ginger tea is used to comfort upset stomachs.

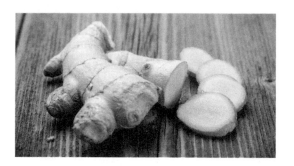

### MEDICINAL PROPERTIES
Analgesic, antiemetic, antiseptic, antispasmodic, bactericidal, carminative, cephalic, expectorant, febrifuge, laxative, rubefacient, stimulant, stomachic, sudorific

### USES
Effective in treating nausea, vomiting, hangovers, and travel sickness; ideal for making pain-relieving salves for sore joints and muscles

### BLENDS WELL WITH
Allspice, anise, Atlas cedarwood, bergamot, cedarwood, clove bud, coriander, eucalyptus (all species), frankincense, galbanum, geranium, grapefruit, jasmine, juniper berry, lemon, lime, mandarin, neroli, palmarosa, patchouli, rose, sweet orange, vetiver, ylang-ylang, yuzu

### PRECAUTIONS
Not recommended for use during pregnancy due to increased risk of skin sensitization. Ginger can cause skin irritation and can be phototoxic; do not apply to skin that will be exposed to direct sunlight.

# GRAPEFRUIT

*Citrus paradisi, C, racemosa,*
*C. maxima var. racemosa*

Sweet, citrus scent
Cost: $

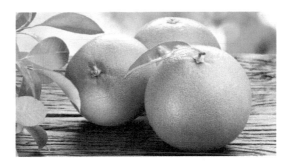

Offering a sweet, tangy, refreshing smell, grapefruit essential oil comes from fresh grapefruit peels. High in vitamin C and valuable to the body's immune system, it offers some protection during cold and flu season. Its diuretic properties make it a valuable ally in the battle against cellulite and water retention, and its uplifting scent provides relief from mental fatigue, depression, and headache.

### MEDICINAL PROPERTIES
Antibacterial, antidepressant, antiseptic, aperitif, astringent, digestive, disinfectant, diuretic, lymphatic stimulant, tonic

### USES
Effective in treating water retention and controlling food cravings

### BLENDS WELL WITH
Bergamot, cardamom, cedarwood, cinnamon leaf, coriander, cypress, davana, ginger, juniper berry, lemon, neroli, palmarosa, peppermint, ravensara leaf, Roman chamomile, rose, sweet orange

### PRECAUTIONS
Phototoxic; do not apply to skin that will be exposed to direct sunlight. Grapefruit can cause sensitive skin. Do not use if taking medications that interact with grapefruit.

# HELICHRYSUM

*Helichrysum italicum*

Strong, herbal scent
Cost: $$$

Helichrysum essential oil isn't cheap, but it is a powerful addition to your aromatherapy arsenal. Sourced from an aromatic evergreen, it is also known as *immortelle,* or everlasting. Traditional uses for this Mediterranean plant include treatments for allergies, colds and coughs, wound healing, indigestion, and much more.

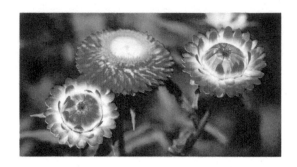

## MEDICINAL PROPERTIES
Analgesic, anti-allergenic, antibacterial, anti-depressant, antifungal, anti-inflammatory, antiseptic, antispasmodic, antitussive, antiviral, astringent, cholagogue, cytophylactic, diuretic, emollient, expectorant, hepatic, nervine, sedative, skin regenerator

## USES
Effective in treating chronic skin conditions, bruises, acne, and arthritis; ideal for making first aid salves and stretch mark balms

## BLENDS WELL WITH
Bergamot, black pepper, clary sage, clove bud, cypress, frankincense, galbanum, geranium, German chamomile, lavender, mandarin, oregano, Roman chamomile, rosewood, sweet orange, tea tree, vetiver, yuzu

## PRECAUTIONS
Generally regarded as safe.

# HOPS FLOWER

*Humulus lupulus*

Spicy, floral scent
Cost: $$$

Hops flowers impart flavor to beers and ales, and are a staple in herbal medicine, where they are revered for their sedative action. Besides helping with insomnia, hops flower essential oil is valuable for easing asthma symptoms and soothing coughs. Applied externally, it is useful for eczema, dandruff, and dry skin.

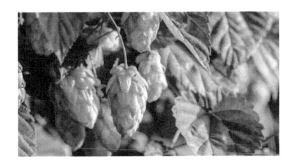

### MEDICINAL PROPERTIES
Analgesic, anti-inflammatory, antispasmodic, antiviral, aphrodisiac, decongestant, relaxant, sedative

### USES
Effective in treating stress, tension, and headaches; ideal for making relaxing bath and body products that nourish skin and hair

### BLENDS WELL WITH
Anise, bergamot, bay laurel, caraway seed, cardamom, cinnamon leaf, clove bud, copaiba, fennel seed, fir needle, ginger, grapefruit, juniper berry, lemon, lime, mandarin, pine, sweet orange, tangerine, yuzu

### PRECAUTIONS
Do not use if clinically depressed. Hops flower can irritate skin.

# HYSSOP

*Hyssopus officinalis*

Sweet, minty, herbal scent
Cost: $$

Hyssop was once nicknamed the "herb of protection" and was used to defend individuals and their homes from malicious influences. In England, it was added to remedies for easing sore muscles and joints. In gardens, its beautiful spikes of violet-blue flowers attract honeybees and other pollinators.

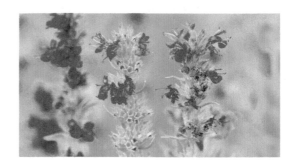

## MEDICINAL PROPERTIES
Antibacterial, antiseptic, antispasmodic, astringent, carminative, cicatrizant, digestive, diuretic, emmenagogue, expectorant, febrifuge, hypertensive, nervine, tonic, vermifuge, vulnerary

## USES
Effective in treating flu and cold symptoms; ideal for making pain-relieving salves for bruises, arthritis, rheumatism, and muscle aches

## BLENDS WELL WITH
Bay laurel, clary sage, geranium, grapefruit, hops flower, lemon, lime, mandarin, melissa, myrtle, rosemary, spearmint, Spanish sage, sweet orange

## PRECAUTIONS
Do not use during pregnancy. Do not use on children less than three years old. Do not use if diagnosed with asthma or epilepsy. Hyssop can cause sensitive skin.

# JASMINE

*Jasminum officinale,*
*J. grandiflorum*

Rich, floral scent
Cost: $$$$

Jasmine absolute is among the most expensive of oils, but a tiny drop goes an incredibly long way. Sourced from star-shaped flowers from a climbing evergreen shrub, jasmine oil begins its journey as a concrete that contains the power of about 1,000 blossoms per pound. From there, absolute is solvent extracted, and essential oil is steam-distilled from the absolute. You can experience the exquisite beauty of jasmine for less by purchasing a blend; many top companies carry pre-diluted jasmine, often with sweet almond oil.

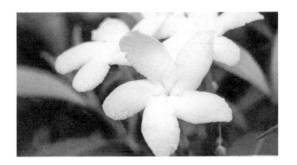

### MEDICINAL PROPERTIES
Analgesic, antidepressant, anti-inflammatory, antiseptic, antispasmodic, aphrodisiac, calmative, carminative, cicatrizant, decongestant, expectorant, galactagogue, parturient, sedative

### USES
Effective in treating impotence, anxiety, depression, and exhaustion; ideal for making personal fragrances and beautifully scented bath and body products

### BLENDS WELL WITH
Clary sage, cypress, frankincense, geranium, lemon, lime, mandarin, rose, rose geranium, rosewood, sandalwood, sweet orange, tangerine, yuzu

### PRECAUTIONS
Do not use during pregnancy. Overuse can cause a headache.

# JUNIPER BERRY

*Juniperus communis*

Fresh, woody scent
Cost: $

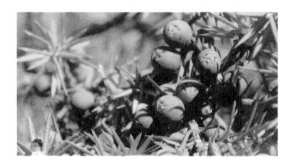

Juniper berries, leaves, and branches have been used for purifying and cleansing the mind, body, and spirit since ancient times, when the trees were believed to ward off illness and negativity while thwarting evil spirits. Native Americans put juniper to good use by making tonics to treat cold, flu, muscle aches, and other ailments, including UTIs.

MEDICINAL PROPERTIES
Antiseptic, antispasmodic, astringent, carminative, depurative, diuretic, rubefacient, stomachic, sudorific, tonic, vulnerary

USES
Effective in treating enlarged prostate, painful periods, gout, arthritis, and rheumatism; ideal for making salves and lotions for treating acne, eczema, psoriasis, oily skin, and dandruff

BLENDS WELL WITH
Atlas cedarwood, bergamot, cedarwood, clary sage, cypress, geranium, grapefruit, lavandin, lavender, lemon, lemongrass, lime, vetiver

PRECAUTIONS
Generally regarded as safe.

# LAVANDIN

*Lavandula latifolia, L. intermedia*

Clean, floral scent
Cost: $

Lavandin is an interesting hybrid plant that was developed in 1900 for use in the perfume and soap-making industry. A cross between true lavender and spike lavender, lavandin is a larger, more productive plant that tolerates colder temperatures than its popular cousin. It is good for easing joint and muscle pain, and it clears lungs and sinuses; like lavender, lavandin is suitable for treating wounds and dermatitis.

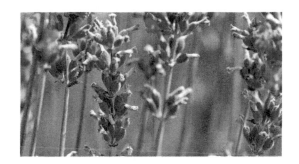

**MEDICINAL PROPERTIES**
Analgesic, antidepressant, antiseptic, anti-spasmodic, cicatrizant, deodorant, diuretic, emmenagogue, expectorant, nervine, sedative, vulnerary

**USES**
Effective in treating cold symptoms and muscle aches; ideal for making fragrant bath and body products

**BLENDS WELL WITH**
Bay laurel, bergamot, cinnamon leaf, clary sage, clove bud, lemongrass, lime, patchouli, pine, rosemary, tangerine, thyme

**PRECAUTIONS**
Do not use during pregnancy.

# LAVENDER
## *Lavandula angustifolia*

Herbaceous, floral scent
Cost: $

Lavender is among the most versatile of all essential oils, thanks to its ability to soothe pain, help wounds heal faster, and ease you into deep, relaxing sleep. Lavender gets its name from the Latin word *lavare,* meaning "to wash," and Romans used it extensively in bathing. It was the Romans who introduced lavender to England, where it remains a favorite today.

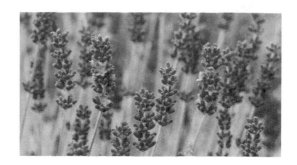

### MEDICINAL PROPERTIES
Analgesic, antidepressant, anti-inflammatory, antiseptic, antispasmodic, antiviral, bactericide, carminative, cholagogue, cicatrizant, cordial, cytophylactic, decongestant, deodorant, diuretic, hypotensive, nervine, rubefacient, sedative, sudorific, vulnerary

### USES
Effective in treating minor burns, cuts, and bruises; ideal for making soothing bedtime bath salts, lotions, and linen sprays

### BLENDS WELL WITH
Atlas cedarwood, cedarwood, clary sage, cypress, galbanum, geranium, juniper berry, lemongrass, melissa, peppermint, pine, rosemary, spearmint, tagetes

### PRECAUTIONS
Generally regarded as safe. Allergic reactions can develop with overuse; discontinue if irritation occurs.

# LEMON

*Citrus limonum*

Sharp, citrus scent
Cost: $

In Japan, lemon essential oil is often diffused in banks and other businesses where sharp attention to detail is required, because the crisp aroma helps promote alertness. Sourced from the same tree that provides tangy, vitamin-rich citrus fruit that goes into popular beverages, candies, and culinary treats, lemon essential oil is a pleasant and useful addition to your aromatherapy kit.

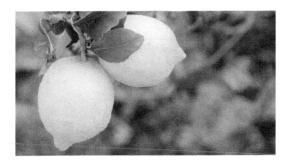

**MEDICINAL PROPERTIES**
Antiseptic, bactericidal, carminative, cicatrizant, depurative, diaphoretic, diuretic, febrifuge, hemostatic, hypotensive, insecticidal, rubefacient, tonic, vermifuge

**USES**
Effective in treating bronchitis, asthma, and respiratory infections; ideal for making bath and body products as well as cleaning products

**BLENDS WELL WITH**
Allspice, benzoin, caraway seed, cardamom, eucalyptus (all types), fennel seed, geranium, juniper berry, neroli, ravensara leaf, ravintsara, rose, rose geranium, rosewood, tagetes

**PRECAUTIONS**
Phototoxic; do not apply to skin that will be exposed to direct sunlight. Lemon can cause sensitive skin.

# LEMON EUCALYPTUS

*Eucalyptus citriodora*

Clean, citrus scent
Cost: $

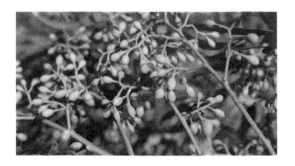

While it offers many of the same properties as other eucalyptus varieties, *Eucalyptus citriodora* has a crisp, lemon scent that some people prefer. Although less potent than *Eucalyptus globulus* and *Eucalyptus radiata,* it is an excellent choice for antiseptic and antifungal use, and its disinfectant qualities make it ideal for using in household cleaners.

## MEDICINAL PROPERTIES
Antibacterial, antidepressant, antifungal, anti-inflammatory, antiseptic, antiviral, expectorant, febrifuge, insect repellent

## USES
Effective in treating congestion, insect bites, and dandruff; ideal for making insect repellent and household cleaners

## BLENDS WELL WITH
Atlas cedarwood, bergamot, cedarwood, cucumber seed, ginger, lavandin, lavender, lemon, lime, marjoram, peppermint, pine, ravensara leaf, rosemary, tea tree

## PRECAUTIONS
Lemon eucalyptus can cause skin irritation.

# LEMON VERBENA

*Lippia citriodora*

Woody, citrus scent
Cost: $$

Offering a gorgeous aroma filled with bright lemon, sensual wood, and fruity, floral undertones, lemon verbena creates a cheerful atmosphere when diffused in your home or office. It calms tension while boosting your spirits, and it offers comfort during periods of digestive distress. Lemon verbena is a potent liver detoxifier, and is useful for dealing with hangovers and overindulgence in rich, fatty foods.

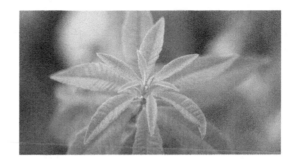

### MEDICINAL PROPERTIES
Antiseptic, antispasmodic, aphrodisiac, digestive, emollient, febrifuge, hepatic, insecticide, sedative, stomachic

### USES
Effective in treating acne, bronchitis, and sinusitis; ideal for making compresses to deal with puffy eyes

### BLENDS WELL WITH
Allspice, davana, elemi, lemon, lime, ginger, mandarin, melissa, palmarosa, yuzu

### PRECAUTIONS
Phototoxic; do not apply to skin that will be exposed to direct sunlight. Lemon verbena can cause sensitive skin.

# LEMONGRASS

*Cymbopogon citratus, C. flexuosus*

Green, citrus scent
Cost: $

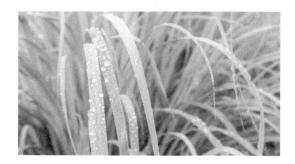

Lemongrass is a popular ingredient in Asian cuisine, and the essential oil often makes its way into natural insect repellents. This aromatic grass is a native of India, where it grows wild and reaches a height of about three feet. There, it is used in Ayurvedic medicine, where it is prized for its ability to treat infections and reduce fevers.

## MEDICINAL PROPERTIES
Analgesic, antidepressant, antimicrobial, antiseptic, astringent, bactericidal, carminative, deodorant, diuretic, febrifuge, fungicidal, galactagogue, insect repellent, insecticidal, nervine

## USES
Effective in treating jet lag, headaches, and stress; ideal for making insect repellent and antifungal bath and body products

## BLENDS WELL WITH
Basil, cajuput, coriander, geranium, jasmine, lavandin, lavender, palmarosa, patchouli, tea tree, vetiver

## PRECAUTIONS
Do not use on children less than two years old. Lemongrass can irritate diseased, damaged, or hypersensitive skin.

# LIME

*Citrus aurantifolia*

Crisp, citrus scent
Cost: $

Originally cultivated in Asia, lime is a delicious citrus fruit that makes its way into beverages, desserts, and more. In the days when sailing ships took months to transport goods from one continent to another, sailors ate limes to prevent scurvy (a condition caused by a severe lack of vitamin C), thus earning the nickname "limeys." Lime essential oil offers a delightful fragrance that adds interest to a variety of aromatherapy blends.

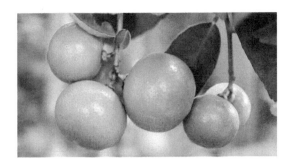

### MEDICINAL PROPERTIES
Antiseptic, antiviral, aperitif, astringent, bactericidal, disinfectant, febrifuge, hemostatic

### USES
Effective in treating painful joints and muscles, respiratory ailments, and acne; ideal for making bath and body products to combat cellulite

### BLENDS WELL WITH
Bergamot, clary sage, juniper berry, lavandin, lavender, lemon, lemon eucalyptus, lemon verbena, lemongrass, neroli, tagetes, ylang-ylang

### PRECAUTIONS
Phototoxic; do not apply to skin that will be exposed to direct sunlight. Lime can cause sensitive skin.

# MANDARIN

*Citrus reticulata*

Sweet, citrus scent
Cost: $

If you are a parent, mandarin is one of the best essential oils to add to your collection. Safe for children and ideal for soothing temper tantrums, it is beautifully uplifting and makes your home smell fantastic. Mandarin is unique from other citrus oils in that it is not phototoxic. Mandarin petit-grain, which comes from the leaves of the same tree that produces mandarin, *is* phototoxic, so be sure not to confuse the two. Sometimes *Citrus reticulata* essential oil is labeled "tangerine." Although the two trees are very closely related, these are two different essential oils. They're quite alike though, so feel free to use them interchangeably.

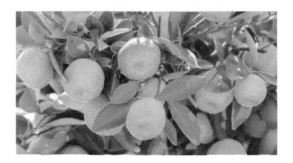

**MEDICINAL PROPERTIES**
Antiseptic, antispasmodic, cytophylactic, depurative, sedative, stomachic, tonic

**USES**
Effective in treating upset stomachs, temper tantrums, and hyperactivity; ideal for making delightfully uplifting bath and body products

**BLENDS WELL WITH**
Allspice, bergamot, clary sage, clove bud, elemi, frankincense, neroli, palo santo, ravensara leaf, tagetes, ylang-ylang

**PRECAUTIONS**
Generally regarded as safe.

# MARJORAM

*Origanum majorana*

Sweet, spicy scent
Cost: $

Also known as sweet marjoram
or knotted marjoram, *Origanum
majorana* originated in North Africa
and the Mediterranean and reached
Egypt sometime around 2000 BCE.
The herb was dedicated to Osiris, the
Egyptian god of the underworld, and it
was used in funerary preparations as
well as in love potions and medicines.
Marjoram is a very relaxing essential
oil, and it's a good choice for cold, flu,
and digestive ailments.

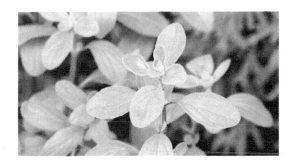

**MEDICINAL PROPERTIES**
Analgesic, antiseptic, antispasmodic, antiviral,
bactericidal, carminative, cephalic, cordial,
diaphoretic, digestive, diuretic, emmenagogue,
expectorant, fungicidal, hypotensive, laxative, nervine, sedative, stomachic, vasodilator,
vulnerary

**USES**
Effective in treating congestion and sinusitis;
ideal for use in warming blends to ease
muscle pain

**BLENDS WELL WITH**
Atlas cedarwood, bergamot, black pepper,
cedarwood, clary sage, cypress, German
chamomile, lavender, lemon, lime, myrtle,
ravensara leaf, Roman chamomile, rosemary,
sweet orange

**PRECAUTIONS**
Do not use during pregnancy.

# MAY CHANG

*Litsea cubeba*

Tropical, fruity scent
Cost: $

Also sold under its botanical name or abbreviated as Litsea, May Chang essential oil offers a delightfully intriguing scent that might make it one of your favorites. This wonderful fragrance comes from a small tree native to China. It has a long history of use for treating ailments ranging from asthma to back pain. Its uplifting fragrance makes it an excellent choice for treating anxiety, fatigue, and depression.

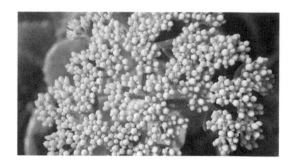

### MEDICINAL PROPERTIES
Antibacterial, antidepressant, anti-inflammatory, antifungal, antiseptic, astringent, deodorant, disinfectant, diuretic, expectorant, insecticide, stimulant, tonic

### USES
Effective in treating chest congestion and indigestion; ideal for making air fresheners, bath and body products, and cleaning products

### BLENDS WELL WITH
Basil, bay laurel, black pepper, cardamom, cedarwood, clary sage, coriander, cypress, davana, eucalyptus (any species), frankincense, geranium, ginger, grapefruit, juniper berry, marjoram, neroli, palmarosa, patchouli, petitgrain, rose, rosemary, rosewood, sandalwood, sweet orange, tea tree, thyme, vetiver, ylang-ylang

### PRECAUTIONS
Not recommended for use during pregnancy due to its ability to increase lactation. May Chang can cause skin irritation.

# MELISSA

*Melissa officinalis*

Sweet, herbal scent
Cost: $$$

Often referred to as lemon balm, melissa essential oil comes from a medicinal herb nicknamed "the elixir of life." A marvelous choice for dealing with stress and tension, melissa reduces blood pressure and settles your nerves. It works wonders for migraines, and can help regulate menstruation while easing associated discomfort.

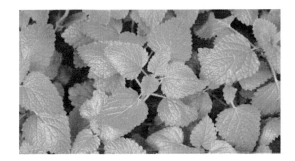

**MEDICINAL PROPERTIES**
Antidepressant, antifungal, antihistaminic, antispasmodic, antiviral, bactericidal, diaphoretic, febrifuge, hypertensive, insect repellent, nervine, sedative, stomachic, sudorific, vermifuge

**USES**
Effective in treating cold sores, cramping, and allergies; ideal for diffusing during times of stress and emotional upset

**BLENDS WELL WITH**
Basil, frankincense, galbanum, geranium, lavender, myrrh, myrtle, peppermint, Roman chamomile, rose, rose geranium, spearmint, ylang-ylang

**PRECAUTIONS**
Melissa can cause skin irritation.

# MYRRH

*Commiphora myrrha*

Warm, woody scent
Cost: $$

Renowned as one of the precious gifts presented to the Christ child by the Magi, myrrh comes from a small tree native to the Middle East and Somalia. Egyptians used it not only as medicine, but employed it in mummification and worship. Myrrh is a wonderful essential oil for skin care, cold and flu season, and diffusing to increase spiritual awareness.

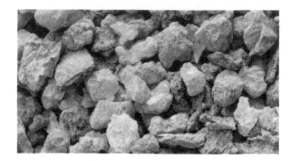

## MEDICINAL PROPERTIES
Anti-inflammatory, antimicrobial, antiseptic, astringent, carminative, cicatrizant, digestive, emmenagogue, expectorant, fungicidal, sedative, stomachic, vulnerary

## USES
Effective in treating sore throats, boils, and chapped skin; ideal for making soothing bath and body products

## BLENDS WELL WITH
Benzoin, bergamot, clove bud, cypress, frankincense, geranium, German chamomile, grapefruit, jasmine, juniper berry, lavender, lemon, lemon eucalyptus, neroli, palmarosa, palo santo, patchouli, pine, Roman chamomile, rose, rosemary, rosewood, sandalwood, tea tree, vetiver, ylang-ylang

## PRECAUTIONS
Do not use during pregnancy.

# MYRTLE

*Myrtus communis*

Light, fresh scent
Cost: $$

Myrtle has long been a representative of peace, love, and harmony; in Britain, it often finds its way into bridal bouquets. Ancient Romans and Greeks valued it for its ability to treat a litany of digestive complaints. Myrtle essential oil addresses a wide range of ailments, yet it is mild enough for young children and seniors.

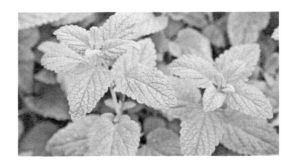

## MEDICINAL PROPERTIES

Antibacterial, antifungal, anti-inflammatory, antimicrobial, antioxidant, antiseptic, antispasmodic, astringent, decongestant, deodorant, digestive, diuretic, emmenagogue, expectorant, laxative, nervine, sedative

## USES

Effective in treating coughs, cold and flu symptoms, and abdominal issues; ideal for making skincare products to sort out acne, psoriasis, and irritation

## BLENDS WELL WITH

Allspice, bay laurel, bergamot, cinnamon leaf, clary sage, clove bud, cypress, ginger, hyssop, lime, melissa, neroli, rosemary

## PRECAUTIONS

Do not use during pregnancy.

# NEROLI

*Citrus aurantium*

Sweet, lingering floral
Cost: $$$$

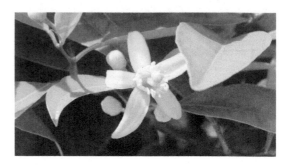

Also known as orange blossom, neroli is extracted from the tiny, white flowers of the bitter orange tree. This extremely relaxing essential oil works well in bedtime blends, and it offers relief from depression, anxiety, and stress. Neroli is an excellent addition to skincare products, as it regenerates skin cells and helps prevent scar tissue. If you find the cost prohibitive but want to enjoy neroli's fragrance, you'll find it is available in fairly inexpensive blends.

## MEDICINAL PROPERTIES
Antidepressant, antiseptic, antispasmodic, aphrodisiac, bactericidal, carminative, cicatrizant, cordial, cytophylactic, deodorant, digestive, emollient, sedative

## USES
Effective in treating insomnia, headaches, and depression; ideal for making lotions to combat stretch marks and scars

## BLENDS WELL WITH
Benzoin, copaiba, cucumber seed, elemi, frankincense, geranium, grapefruit, lavender, lemon, lime, jasmine, mandarin, palo santo, petitgrain, rosemary, rosewood, sandalwood, spikenard, yuzu

## PRECAUTIONS
Neroli can be very relaxing; be aware of how it affects you before driving or undertaking important tasks.

# NIAOULI

*Melaleuca quinquenervia,*
*var. cineole*

Fresh, sweet scent
Cost: $

Niaouli is closely related to tea tree, and although it is milder, it shares many of the same characteristics. A native of Australia, the niaouli tree's leaves were historically made into poultices for treating fevers, aching joints, and headaches. Niaouli has the ability to enhance the body's immune response, and is an excellent choice for respiratory illnesses.

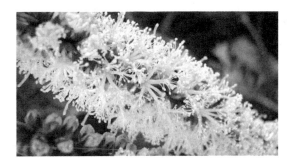

### MEDICINAL PROPERTIES
Analgesic, antibacterial, antiseptic, antispasmodic, decongestant, expectorant, febrifuge, insecticide, vermifuge, vulnerary

### USES
Effective in treating bronchitis, asthma, sinusitis, and laryngitis; ideal for making first aid salves to treat minor cuts, burns, and insect bites

### BLENDS WELL WITH
Clary sage, clove bud, coriander, eucalyptus (any species), fennel seed, juniper berry, lavender, lime, peppermint, pine, rosemary, spearmint

### PRECAUTIONS
Generally regarded as safe.

# OREGANO

*Origanum vulgare*

Spicy, herbaceous scent
Cost: $$

While some sources decry oregano as too powerful an oil to use in aromatherapy, it offers a number of medicinal properties, and can be of great benefit when used with a careful hand. The herb itself is potent; ancient Greeks used oregano leaves on sore, aching muscles and wounds, and early European herbalists recommended it as a digestive aid.

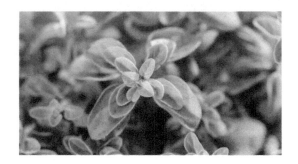

### MEDICINAL PROPERTIES
Analgesic, anthelmintic, antibacterial, antifungal, anti-inflammatory, antiseptic, antispasmodic, antitoxic, antiviral, carminative, disinfectant, diuretic, emmenagogue, expectorant

### USES
Effective in treating warts and sinus infections; ideal for use in insect repellents

### BLENDS WELL WITH
Cypress, German chamomile, lavender, marjoram, pine, Roman chamomile, rosemary

### PRECAUTIONS
Do not use during pregnancy. Do not use on children less than 10 years old. Oregano can cause severe skin irritation.

# PALMAROSA

*Cymbopogon martinii*

Sweet, floral scent
Cost: $

While palmarosa is sometimes referred to as Turkish or East Indian geranium, it comes from a wild-growing grass with straw-colored leaves and flowering tops. Despite its floral scent, the herb is harvested before the flowers appear. Palmarosa is used commercially to scent tobacco, soaps, cosmetics, and perfumes.

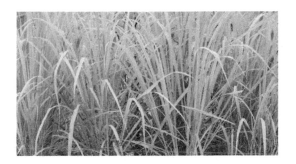

### MEDICINAL PROPERTIES
Analgesic, antiseptic, antiviral, bactericide, cicatrizant, cytophylactic, digestive, febrifuge

### USES
Effective in treating digestive issues, cold, and flu; ideal for making nourishing skincare blends that address acne and dermatitis while regenerating skin

### BLENDS WELL WITH
Bergamot, geranium, lemon, lime, mandarin, melissa, neroli, patchouli, petitgrain, ravensara leaf, rose, rose geranium, rosemary, rosewood, sweet orange, tangerine, ylang-ylang, yuzu

### PRECAUTIONS
Generally regarded as safe.

# PALO SANTO

*Bursera graveolens*

Sweet, woody scent
Cost: $$

If you like frankincense, you're likely to appreciate palo santo. This oil offers a calming, grounding presence that eases anxiety, depression, and emotional upset, and a tiny drop goes a long way. In Ecuador and Peru, where "holy wood" is grown, the smoke is used to keep flying insects at bay and treat respiratory ailments.

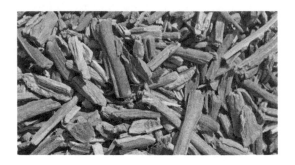

**MEDICINAL PROPERTIES**
Antidepressant, anti-inflammatory, calmative, deodorant, insect repellent, relaxant

**USES**
Effective in treating irritated skin and joint soreness; ideal for creating a peaceful, meditative atmosphere in your home

**BLENDS WELL WITH**
Atlas cedarwood, bergamot, cedarwood, davana, frankincense, helichrysum, mandarin, myrrh, neroli, patchouli, rose, rosewood, sandalwood, vetiver, ylang-ylang

**PRECAUTIONS**
Generally regarded as safe.

# PATCHOULI

*Pogostemon cablin*

Sweet, spicy, woody scent
Cost: $$

Arguably one of the most intriguing
of scents, patchouli became popular
when textile companies began using
it to repel lice and fleas in fabric
used to make clothing and bedding.
It was also used to give India ink
its signature smell. Patchouli has a
long history of masking unpleasant
odors and serving as a base note in
perfumes; despite its popularity in
aromatic applications, it offers a
wide range of medicinal properties.

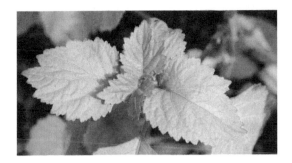

MEDICINAL PROPERTIES
Antidepressant, antiemetic, antifungal,
anti-inflammatory, antimicrobial, antiseptic,
antiviral, aphrodisiac, astringent, calmative,
carminative, cicatrizant, deodorant, digestive,
diuretic, febrifuge, fungicidal, insect repellent,
insecticide, sedative

USES
Effective in treating hemorrhoids, yeast
infections, and fungal infections, including
athlete's foot; ideal for use in perfumes and
skincare products

BLENDS WELL WITH
Bergamot, clary sage, davana, geranium,
lavender, mandarin, myrrh, palmarosa, rose
geranium, Spanish sage, spikenard, sweet
orange, tangerine, yuzu

PRECAUTIONS
Generally regarded as safe.

# PEPPERMINT

*Mentha piperita*

Crisp, minty
Cost: $

Peppermint has been cultivated
throughout human history, with
evidence of its use being found in
an Egyptian tomb that dates back to
1000 BCE. Greek mythology describes
peppermint's origin as the result
of an act of jealousy: Pluto's envious
wife, Persephone, trod a nymph
called Mentha into the ground in
a fit of rage. Pluto transformed
Mentha into an herb for people
to enjoy for eternity.

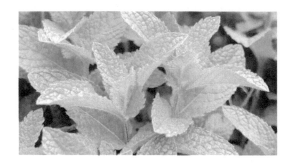

MEDICINAL PROPERTIES
Analgesic, anti-inflammatory, antiseptic, antispasmodic, astringent, carminative, cephalic,
cholagogue, cordial, decongestant, emmenagogue, expectorant, febrifuge, hepatic, nervine,
stimulant, stomachic, sudorific, vasoconstrictor,
vermifuge

USES
Effective in treating headaches and indigestion;
ideal for making comforting salves to treat sunburn, itching, and skin inflammation

BLENDS WELL WITH
Benzoin, eucalyptus (any species), fir needle,
German chamomile, juniper berry, lavender,
lemon, mandarin, marjoram, melissa, niaouli,
pine, ravintsara, rosemary, tangerine

PRECAUTIONS
Do not use during pregnancy. Not recommended for use on children less than six years
old. Peppermint can cause skin irritation and
irritate mucous membranes.

# PETITGRAIN

*Citrus aurantium*

Fresh, slightly bitter floral scent
Cost: $

Often referred to as "poor man's neroli" because the two oils are interchangeable in many instances, petitgrain is an outstanding anti-depressant that is ideal for easing mild, long-term disorders, including seasonal affective disorder (SAD). It stimulates clear thinking, relieves stress, and eliminates brain fog. If you blend petitgrain, neroli, and bergamot together, you'll be enjoying three unique essential oils from the same tree, all at the same time.

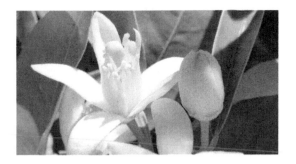

**MEDICINAL PROPERTIES**
Antidepressant, antiseptic, antispasmodic, deodorant, digestive, nervine, sedative, stomachic

**USES**
Effective in treating respiratory infections, asthma, and congestion; ideal for making uplifting bath and body products that promote balanced skin

**BLENDS WELL WITH**
Atlas cedarwood, balsam of Peru, bergamot, black pepper, cedarwood, clove bud, coriander, cypress, elemi, frankincense, mandarin, May Chang, neroli, patchouli, rose, rosewood, sweet orange, tangerine, vetiver, yuzu

**PRECAUTIONS**
Generally regarded as safe.

# PINE

*Pinus sylvestris*

Fresh, green-forest scent
Cost: $

While many think of pine simply as a source of wood, it has been used for many things throughout history. Native Americans and others used its rich, delicious seeds as an important source of protein and fat, and employed its needles as a source of vitamin C to prevent scurvy. Among its many medicinal uses are relief from arthritis, muscle, and joint pain, and the treatment of respiratory illnesses.

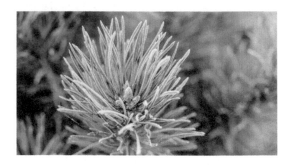

## MEDICINAL PROPERTIES
Analgesic, antibacterial, antiseptic, antiviral, cholagogue, deodorant, diuretic, expectorant, insecticide, rubefacient, stimulant, sudorific, vermifuge

## USES
Effective in treating cold, cough, sinusitis, and bronchitis; ideal for making soothing salves to ease muscle and joint pain

## BLENDS WELL WITH
Atlas cedarwood, bay laurel, cedarwood, clary sage, eucalyptus (all species), fir needle, juniper, lavender, lemon, niaouli, ravensara leaf, rosemary, Spanish sage, spikenard

## PRECAUTIONS
Not recommended for use during pregnancy due to the increased risk of skin sensitization. Pine can cause skin irritation.

# RAVENSARA LEAF

*Ravensara aromatica,*
*Agathophyllum aromatica*

Fruity, slightly medicinal scent
Cost: $

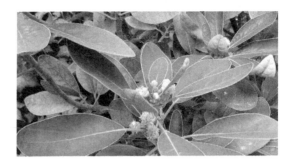

Ravensara leaf comes from Madagascar, where it is believed to be a cure-all in much the same way that tea tree is esteemed in Australia. It is a good choice for pain relief, including headaches, muscle and joint soreness, toothache, and earache. Some sources confuse ravensara leaf with ravintsara. Although the two species have similar-sounding names, they offer very different properties.

**MEDICINAL PROPERTIES**
Analgesic, anti-allergenic, antibacterial, antidepressant, antifungal, antiseptic, antispasmodic, antiviral, aphrodisiac, disinfectant, diuretic, expectorant, relaxant

**USES**
Effective in treating minor wounds, water retention, eczema, and shingles; ideal for diffusing to ease stress, nervousness, and insomnia

**BLENDS WELL WITH**
Atlas cedarwood, bay laurel, bergamot, black pepper, cardamom, cedarwood, clary sage, cypress, eucalyptus (any species), frankincense, geranium, ginger, grapefruit, lavender, lemon, mandarin, marjoram, palmarosa, pine, rosemary, rosewood, sandalwood, tea tree, thyme

**PRECAUTIONS**
Do not use during pregnancy. Ravensara leaf can cause skin irritation.

# RAVINTSARA

*Cinnamomum camphora*

Earthy, fresh scent
Cost: $$

Often referred to as Ho wood, ravintsara essential oil comes from the root stumps, wood, and branches of a tree traditionally used to craft handles for Japanese knives and swords. Today, the wood is often used to build cabinets and architectural trim pieces. In China, statues of Buddha are often carved from Ho wood.

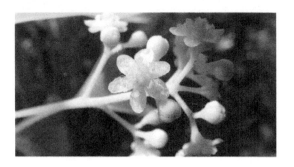

### MEDICINAL PROPERTIES
Antibacterial, antifungal, anti-inflammatory, antiseptic, antispasmodic, antiviral, carminative, diuretic, expectorant, stimulant

### USES
Effective in treating cold sores, chicken pox, shingles, and viral infections; ideal for diffusing and vaporizing to treat respiratory illnesses

### BLENDS WELL WITH
Basil, cajuput, German chamomile, helichrysum, lavender, lemon, peppermint, Roman chamomile, rosewood, sandalwood, spearmint, ylang-ylang

### PRECAUTIONS
Ravintsara can cause skin irritation.

# ROMAN CHAMOMILE

*Anthemis nobilis*

Sweet, herbal scent
Cost: $$$

Roman chamomile offers a pleasant scent that reminds many people of ripe apples. In aromatherapy, it is highly prized for its skin-healing properties and its ability to calm frayed nerves. If you suffer from PMS or are feeling irritable or impatient, this is an excellent oil to try.

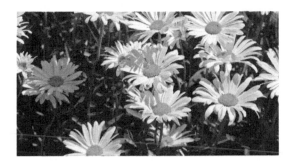

**MEDICINAL PROPERTIES**
Analgesic, antibiotic, antidepressant, anti-inflammatory, antiseptic, antispasmodic, bactericidal, carminative, cholagogue, cicatrizant, digestive, emmenagogue, febrifuge, hepatic, nervine, sedative, stomachic, sudorific, tonic, vermifuge, vulnerary

**USES**
Effective in treating dry, chapped skin, infant teething, acne, eczema, and dermatitis; ideal in blends for alleviating indigestion and colic

**BLENDS WELL WITH**
Bergamot, cajuput, carrot seed, clary sage, cucumber seed, elemi, eucalyptus (any species), frankincense, geranium, grapefruit, jasmine, lavender, lemon, neroli, palmarosa, rose, rose geranium, rosewood, tea tree

**PRECAUTIONS**
Do not use during pregnancy. Roman chamomile can cause skin irritation.

# ROSE

*Rosa damascena*

Sweet, floral scent
Cost: $$$$

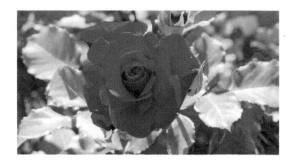

Inside each bottle of pure rose oil, you'll find the power of more than 1,000 roses, all picked at the peak of their potency. A little drop goes a long way, helping prevent scarring, rejuvenating aging or dry skin, and soothing the discomfort of eczema, shingles, and other painful disorders. If you find the cost of pure rose or rose otto prohibitive, but want to experience the fragrance, you'll find that many top retailers offer delightful pre-diluted rose oils for a fraction of the cost.

## MEDICINAL PROPERTIES
Antidepressant, anti-inflammatory, antiseptic, antispasmodic, antiviral, aphrodisiac, astringent, bactericidal, cicatrizant, depurative, emmenagogue, hemostatic, hepatic, laxative

## USES
Effective in treating impotence, depression, anger, and stress; ideal for making soothing bath and body products

## BLENDS WELL WITH
Balsam of Peru, bergamot, clove bud, davana, frankincense, galbanum, geranium, jasmine, melissa, myrrh, palmarosa, patchouli, rosewood, yuzu

## PRECAUTIONS
Do not use during pregnancy.

# ROSE GERANIUM

*Pelargonium graveolens*

Green, floral scent
Cost: $$

Sometimes referred to as bourbon geranium, rose geranium has a light, rosy scent with minty undertones. Rose geranium's ability to stimulate the adrenal cortex (the outer part of the adrenal gland) makes it useful in lifting depression and alleviating anxiety. It stimulates the lymph system to aid in detoxification, and it helps balance dry and oily skin.

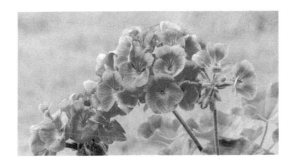

**MEDICINAL PROPERTIES**
Antidepressant, antiseptic, astringent, cicatrizant, cytophylactic, deodorant, diuretic, hemostatic, styptic, vermifuge, vulnerary

**USES**
Effective in treating sunburn, PMS, and painful periods; ideal for making nourishing bath and body products

**BLENDS WELL WITH**
Basil, bergamot, carrot seed, cedarwood, citronella, clary sage, cucumber seed, grapefruit, jasmine, lavender, lemon, lime, mandarin, neroli, patchouli, rosemary, sweet orange

**PRECAUTIONS**
Not recommend for use during pregnancy due to rose geranium's hormone-balancing properties.

# ROSEMARY

*Rosmarinus officinalis*

Refreshing, herbal scent
Cost: $

Rosemary has the intriguing ability to stimulate memory and facilitate clear thinking. In ancient Greece, scholars wore rosemary while studying, as it helped them retain information. Diffusing rosemary essential oil can sharpen your focus and aid with productivity while promoting a sense of calm confidence.

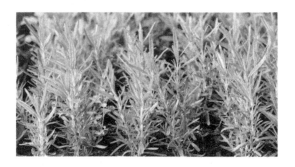

### MEDICINAL PROPERTIES
Analgesic, antibacterial, antidepressant, antifungal, antimicrobial, antioxidant, antiseptic, antispasmodic, astringent, carminative, cicatrizant, digestive, diuretic, emmenagogue, hepatic, hypertensive, stimulant, sudorific, vulnerary

### USES
Effective in treating digestive complaints, muscle pain, thinning hair, and dandruff; ideal for making bath and body products to balance skin and nourish hair

### BLENDS WELL WITH
Balsam of Peru, basil, bay laurel, bergamot, cajuput, clary sage, clove bud, elemi, fennel seed, juniper berry, lemon, niaouli, peppermint, petitgrain, Spanish sage, spearmint, tea tree

### PRECAUTIONS
Do not use during pregnancy. Do not use if diagnosed with epilepsy. Rosemary is quite stimulating; using it within three to four hours of bedtime can cause wakefulness.

# ROSEWOOD

*Aniba rosaeodora*

Spicy, woody scent
Cost: $$

Also known as Pau-Rosa, Brazilian rosewood, or bois de rose, rosewood essential oil comes from the wood of the Brazilian rosewood tree, which is endangered in the wild. When shopping for this beautiful, nourishing oil, be sure to select one that is ethically harvested from a rosewood farm. These managed plantations provide rosewood for carving and furniture making, and are careful to plant more trees than they harvest.

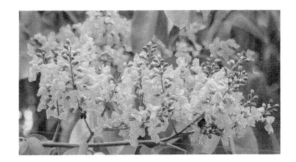

### MEDICINAL PROPERTIES
Analgesic, antibacterial, antidepressant, antimicrobial, antiseptic, aphrodisiac, calmative, deodorant, emollient, euphoriant, stimulant

### USES
Effective in treating dry, chapped skin; ideal for making nourishing bath and body products that lift the spirits

### BLENDS WELL WITH
Benzoin, bergamot, clary sage, copaiba, davana, jasmine, lavender, lemon, mandarin, May Chang, neroli, palmarosa, petitgrain, rose, sweet orange, tangerine, vetiver, ylang-ylang, yuzu

### PRECAUTIONS
Generally regarded as safe.

# SANDALWOOD

*Santalum album*

Sweet, woody scent
Cost: $$$$

Sandalwood essential oil comes from the dead roots and wood of very old *Santalum album* trees. Prized as a perfume material since ancient times, it is also used in incense sticks and for making furniture. Like rosewood, sandalwood is subject to poaching and improper harvesting; however, most well-known essential oil companies take care to source their product ethically, from farmers who raise the trees.

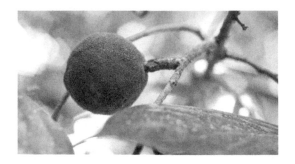

MEDICINAL PROPERTIES
Antidepressant, anti-inflammatory, antiseptic, antispasmodic, aphrodisiac, astringent, carminative, cicatrizant, digestive, diuretic, expectorant, insect repellent, nervine, sedative, stomachic, tonic, vermifuge, vulnerary

USES
Effective in treating psoriasis, eczema, and dry skin; ideal for diffusing to create an enticing, romantic atmosphere

BLENDS WELL WITH
Bergamot, black pepper, geranium, jasmine, lavender, myrrh, neroli, rose, vetiver, ylang-ylang, yuzu

PRECAUTIONS
Generally regarded as safe. Sandalwood essential oil gets stronger over time; a tiny drop goes a long way.

# SPANISH SAGE

*Salvia lavandulaefolia*

Strong, herbaceous scent
Cost: $$

Spanish sage is among a few different types of essential oil marketed as "sage," and is not to be confused with Dalmatian sage (*Salvia officinalis*). It is a very potent oil that calls for a light, judicious hand, but it proves effective as a mood lifter, memory aid, and remedy for dealing with PMS, painful periods, and menopause symptoms.

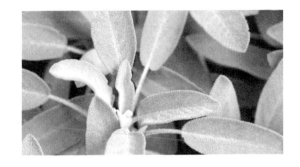

## MEDICINAL PROPERTIES
Anti-inflammatory, antimicrobial, antioxidant, antiseptic, emmenagoque

## USES
Effective in treating hot flashes, night sweats, insomnia; ideal for adding to salves for easing aches and pains

## BLENDS WELL WITH
Bergamot, lavender, lemon, lime, sweet orange, rosewood, sandalwood

## PRECAUTIONS
Do not use during pregnancy or breastfeeding. Do not use if diagnosed with epilepsy or high blood pressure.

# SPEARMINT

*Mentha spicata, M. viridis*

Sweet, minty scent
Cost: $

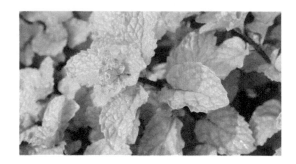

A gentler substitute for peppermint essential oil, spearmint calms itching, relieves coughs and colds, eases indigestion, and has a marvelously uplifting effect on the mind. A Mediterranean native that is now cultivated worldwide, spearmint was used by ancient Greeks, who enjoyed the scent in their bath water. During medieval times, it was used to whiten teeth and soothe sore gums, much in the way we use fresh, minty toothpaste today.

## MEDICINAL PROPERTIES
Antidepressant, antiseptic, antispasmodic, astringent, carminative, cephalic, decongestant, digestive, diuretic, expectorant, insecticide, stimulant, stomachic

## USES
Effective in treating halitosis, hiccups, and headaches; ideal for making balms to treat acne and itching

## BLENDS WELL WITH
Basil, bay laurel, benzoin, eucalyptus (any species), jasmine, lavender, lemon, lime, mandarin, niaouli, peppermint, rosemary, sweet orange, tangerine

## PRECAUTIONS
Do not use spearmint if breastfeeding, as it can reduce lactation. Spearmint is unique in that it can sometimes weaken homeopathic remedies; if you take a homeopathic remedy, ensure that spearmint is compatible before using it.

# SPIKENARD
### *Nardostachys jatamansi*

Musky, woody scent
Cost: $$$

A favorite of ancient Egyptians, spikenard was also mentioned in the Bible's Song of Solomon as well as in the Book of John. It was often used to make tea for treating nervousness and heart palpitations, and in India, Ayurvedic practitioners use it to aid healthy liver function. Spikenard essential oil is sometimes called false valerian: Like the real thing, it can promote deep, restful sleep.

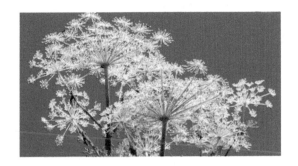

**MEDICINAL PROPERTIES**
Antibacterial, antifungal, anti-inflammatory, antioxidant, antiseptic, antispasmodic, deodorant, digestive, diuretic, febrifuge, laxative, sedative

**USES**
Effective in treating insomnia, stress, and nervousness; ideal for making bath and body products to soothe and nourish dry or aging skin

**BLENDS WELL WITH**
Cardamom, cinnamon leaf, clary sage, coriander, fennel seed, lavender, neroli, patchouli, pine, vetiver

**PRECAUTIONS**
Not recommended for use during pregnancy due to spikenard's deeply relaxing effect. Do not use on children less than six years old.

# SPRUCE

*Picea mariana*

Fresh, forest scent
Cost: $

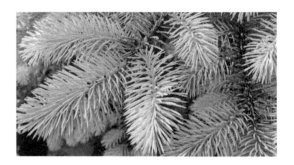

Also known as black spruce, *Picea mariana* is a slow-growing coniferous tree that is part of the pine family. The provincial tree of Labrador and Newfoundland, it is native to North America's boreal forests. There are a few other spruce oils on the market with similar properties, but black spruce offers the sweetest, lightest aroma among them.

## MEDICINAL PROPERTIES
Anti-inflammatory, antiseptic, antispasmodic, antitussive, astringent, diuretic, expectorant, nervine, vulnerary

## USES
Effective in colds, coughs, flu, and respiratory ailments; ideal for making warming salves to treat joint and muscle pain

## BLENDS WELL WITH
Atlas cedarwood, benzoin, cedarwood, clary sage, cypress, eucalyptus (any species), fir needle, frankincense, galbanum, lavender, lemon, palo santo, petitgrain, pine, rose, rosemary, rosewood, sandalwood

## PRECAUTIONS
Spruce gets stronger with age; it can cause skin sensitization when oxidized. Use up within six months of opening for topical use, and reserve older oil for inhalation and household cleaning purposes.

# SWEET ORANGE

*Citrus sinensis*

Sweet, citrus scent
Cost: $

Oranges make a fantastic snack, but historically, they have also been put to medicinal and cosmetic uses. In ancient China, dried oranges were a popular remedy for a bloated stomach, and the peel was used to relieve coughing. Sweet orange's enticing aroma is good for more than just air fresheners; it (and other citrus oils) have been successfully used it to curb cigarette cravings.

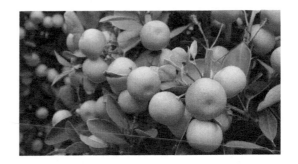

### MEDICINAL PROPERTIES
Antibacterial, antidepressant, anti-inflammatory, antiseptic, antiviral, aperitif, astringent, carminative, cholagogue, digestive, diuretic, fungicidal, hypotensive, stomachic, tonic

### USES
Effective in treating cold, flu, and digestive ailments; ideal for making air fresheners and cleaning products

### BLENDS WELL WITH
Anise, allspice, black pepper, caraway seed, cardamom, cinnamon leaf, clove bud, copaiba, elemi, fennel seed, frankincense, galbanum, ginger, rosewood, sandalwood, tagetes, vetiver

### PRECAUTIONS
Phototoxic: Do not apply to skin that will be exposed to direct sunlight. Use up within six months of opening for topical use, and reserve older oil for inhalation and household cleaning purposes.

# TAGETES

*Tagetes minuta*

Sharp, green herbal scent
Cost: $

Sometimes referred to as marigold or Mexican marigold, tagetes is not to be confused with calendula. A very strong insect repellent and insecticide, tagetes is native to Africa, where it can sometimes be seen hanging in bunches to deter mosquitoes and flies. Also known as khaki bush, tagetes is now grown throughout France and North America, where it is popular with the perfume industry.

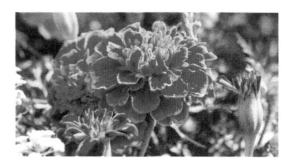

MEDICINAL PROPERTIES
Antibiotic, antimicrobial, antiseptic, antispasmodic, insect repellent, insecticide, sedative

USES
Effective in treating cough, cold, and bronchitis; ideal for making insect repellents

BLENDS WELL WITH
Bergamot, clary sage, jasmine, lavender, lemon, lime, mandarin, neroli, sweet orange

PRECAUTIONS
Not recommended for use during pregnancy due to the risk of skin sensitization. Tagetes can cause skin irritation, particularly in those with sensitive skin. Phototoxic: Do not apply to skin that will be exposed to direct sunlight.

# TANGERINE

*Citrus reticulata blanco*

Sweet, citrus scent
Cost: $

Tangerine is closely related to mandarin essential oil, and the two are often used interchangeably despite subtle differences in fragrance. Tangerine's aroma is sweeter and a bit heavier than that of mandarin, which is light and almost candy-like. Both bring feelings of joy and relieve stress, and both are ideal for use around children. Like mandarin, tangerine is not typically phototoxic.

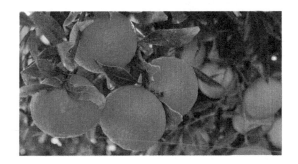

**MEDICINAL PROPERTIES**
Antiseptic, antispasmodic, cytophylactic, depurative, sedative, stomachic, tonic

**USES**
Effective in treating stress, nervousness, and depression; ideal for making air fresheners and scented bath and body products

**BLENDS WELL WITH**
Allspice, bergamot, caraway seed, cardamom, clary sage, clove bud, elemi, frankincense, ginger, myrrh, neroli, ylang-ylang

**PRECAUTIONS**
Generally regarded as safe.

# TEA TREE

*Melaleuca alternifolia*

Light, camphor scent
Cost: $

One of the most potent immune-stimulating essential oils available, tea tree comes from New South Wales in Australia, where aboriginal people first enjoyed its many medicinal purposes. During World War II, tea tree was so important to the Allies that tea tree cutters and producers were exempt from military service. Soldiers and sailors used it the same way as it is employed today—to treat minor wounds, infections, and more.

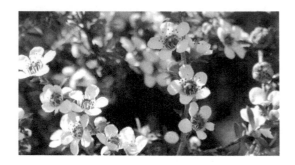

### MEDICINAL PROPERTIES
Antimicrobial, antiseptic, antiviral, bactericide, cicatrizant, expectorant, fungicide, insect repellent, insecticide, stimulant, sudorific

### USES
Effective in treating minor wounds, sinusitis, and respiratory ailments; ideal for making powerful antiseptic household cleaners

### BLENDS WELL WITH
Cinnamon leaf, clary sage, clove bud, eucalyptus (any species), geranium, lavender, lemon, myrrh, oregano, rosemary, rosewood, thyme

### PRECAUTIONS
Generally regarded as safe.

# THYME

*Thymus vulgaris*

Spicy, herbaceous scent
Cost: $$

Thyme has a long history of culinary use, as well as an interesting medicinal background. Ancient Greeks used it to repel insects, and Romans believed bathing in thyme-scented water would impart courage and vigor. Thyme is a spicy oil that must be used judiciously. In salves and compresses, it increases circulation, making it ideal for treating sprains, bruises, and muscle aches.

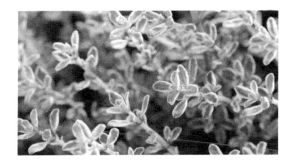

## MEDICINAL PROPERTIES
Antibacterial, antifungal, antimicrobial, antioxidant, antiseptic, antispasmodic, antitoxic, antitussive, astringent, cicatrizant, disinfectant, expectorant, hypertensive, insect repellent, insecticide, stimulant, sudorific

## USES
Effective in treating diarrhea, infectious colitis, and upper respiratory infections; ideal for making insect repellents

## BLENDS WELL WITH
Balsam of Peru, bay laurel, bergamot, black pepper, clary sage, fir needle, grapefruit, juniper berry, lemon, lime, lavender, pine, rosemary, Spanish sage

## PRECAUTIONS
Do not use on children less than six years old.

# VALERIAN

*Valerian officinalis*

Complex musky scent
Cost: $$

Valerian's power to calm the central nervous system comes from two sesquiterpenes: valerone and valerenic acid. A drop or two of this potent essential oil applied to the feet or temples promotes sound, refreshing sleep, just as do herbal sleep aids containing valerian.

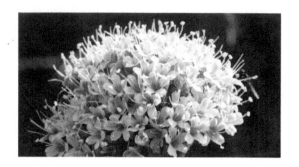

### MEDICINAL PROPERTIES
Antispasmodic, bactericidal, carminative, diuretic, hypnotic, hypotensive, nervous system depressant, sedative

### USES
Effective in treating insomnia, nervous tension, and exhaustion; ideal for making calming bath and body products

### BLENDS WELL WITH
Atlas cedarwood, cedarwood, clary sage, lavender, mandarin, patchouli, petitgrain, pine, rose, rosemary, rosewood, sandalwood, tangerine

### PRECAUTIONS
Do not use during pregnancy. Do not use with antidepressants, pharmaceutical sedatives, or alcohol.

# VETIVER

*Chrysopogon zizanioides*

Sweet, woody scent
Cost: $

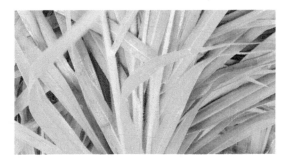

Vetiver is a tufted, perennial grass native to the tropics, where it is used to weave fragrant mats, baskets, and window coverings, and also for erosion control in wet areas. Besides its many practical uses, vetiver is widely employed by the fragrance industry. In aromatherapy, it is called the "oil of tranquility" for its ability to ward off depression while calming nervousness and stress.

### MEDICINAL PROPERTIES
Analgesic, anti-inflammatory, antiseptic, antispasmodic, aphrodisiac, astringent, calmative, cicatrizant, detoxifier, insect repellent, nervine, sedative, stomachic, tonic, vulnerary

### USES
Effective in treating ADHD, stress, and postpartum depression; ideal for making soothing products to ease the pain of arthritis, rheumatism, muscle strains, and more

### BLENDS WELL WITH
Benzoin, cardamom, clary sage, fennel seed, grapefruit, jasmine, mandarin, marjoram, May Chang, neroli, patchouli, petitgrain, sweet orange, tangerine, ylang-ylang

### PRECAUTIONS
Generally regarded as safe.

# VITEX BERRY

*Vitex agnus-castus*

Minty herbal scent with berry undertones
Cost: $$$

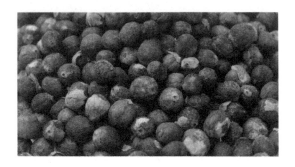

Also known as chaste tree, chaste-berry, or monk's pepper, vitex berry has a long traditional use as a hormone balancer, particularly for those who are suffering from PMS, painful periods, or menopause symptoms. It has a progesterone-like effect on the body and must be used in small increments.

## MEDICINAL PROPERTIES
Anaphrodisiac, diaphoretic, diuretic, emmenagogue, febrifuge, galactagogue, sedative, vulnerary

## USES
Effective in treating cramps, breast tenderness, and depression associated with PMS; ideal for making treatments for period-related acne and easing turbulent emotions

## BLENDS WELL WITH
Clary sage, geranium, lavender, May Chang, rose, rose geranium, valerian

## PRECAUTIONS
Do not use during pregnancy. Do not use in conjunction with birth control pills or hormone-replacement therapies. Do not use on children.

# YLANG-YLANG

*Cananga odorata*

Sweet floral scent
Cost: $$

Sometimes referred to as "poor man's jasmine," ylang-ylang has a beautifully haunting scent that makes it a favorite with perfumeries. Pronounced *ee-lang ee-lang*, ylang ylang means "flower of flowers." Like jasmine, neroli, and other heady florals, a little bit goes a long way.

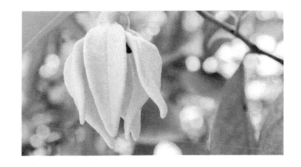

**MEDICINAL PROPERTIES**
Antidepressant, antiseborrheic, antiseptic, aphrodisiac, hypotensive, nervine, sedative

**USES**
Effective in treating stress, nervousness, and anxiety; ideal for making romantic, relaxing bath and body products

**BLENDS WELL WITH**
Bergamot, cypress, davana, grapefruit, lavender, lemon, mandarin, petitgrain, rosewood, sandalwood, tangerine, vetiver, yuzu

**PRECAUTIONS**
Generally regarded as safe; however, overuse can cause nausea and headaches.

# YUZU

*Citrus junos*

Floral citrus scent
Cost: $$$

Yuzu is a citrus fruit that is very popular in Japan, where it is made into marmalade, blended into ice cream, and enjoyed whole. The aromatic rinds are sometimes added to a hot bath, where they are used to refresh the mind and ward off colds and the flu. Yuzu is an excellent oil to diffuse when you're feeling stressed, burned out, or frustrated.

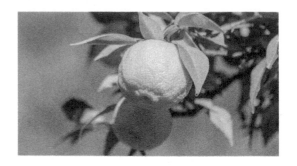

## MEDICINAL PROPERTIES
Antidepressant, antiseptic, antispasmodic, calmative, cicatrizant, deodorant, digestive, febrifuge, vulnerary

## USES
Effective in treating cold and flu; ideal for blending personal fragrances and making uplifting bath and body products

## BLENDS WELL WITH
Basil, benzoin, clary sage, cypress, davana, frankincense, ginger, jasmine, neroli, patchouli, petitgrain, palmarosa, rose, rosewood, sandalwood, vetiver, ylang-ylang

## PRECAUTIONS
Phototoxic: Do not apply to skin that will be exposed to direct sunlight.

# MEASUREMENT CONVERSIONS

Due to differences in utensils, variation in drop size, and differences in user judgment, these measurement conversions are approximate. You will find some of these measurements in this book; others are found in other aromatherapy resources.

| |
|---|
| 1 ml = 20 drops = 0.03 ounce = 0.27 dram |
| 15 ml = 0.5 ounce = ½ ounce |
| 1 teaspoon = 1 dram = 75 drops = ⅛ ounce = 3.7 ml |
| 3 teaspoons = 1 tablespoon |
| 2 tablespoons = 1 ounce |
| 16 tablespoons = 8 ounces = 1 cup |
| 2 cups = 1 pint |
| 4 cups = 1 quart |
| 4 quarts = 1 gallon |

# GLOSSARY

**adulterate:** to mix pure essential oils with less expensive substances, but advertise the product as 100% pure essential oil.

**analgesic:** a substance that relieves or deadens pain.

**anaphrodisiac:** a substance that reduces sexual desire.

**anesthetic:** a substance that relieves pain via loss of sensation.

**anti-allergenic:** a substance that reduces allergy symptoms.

**antibacterial:** a substance that fights bacterial growth.

**antibiotic:** a substance that fights infections by destroying bacteria in the body, or by preventing bacterial growth within the body.

**antidepressant:** a substance that elevates the mood and counteracts depression.

**antiemetic:** a substance that reduces the severity or frequency of vomiting.

**antifungal:** a substance that prevents fungal growth.

**anti-inflammatory:** a substance that reduces or prevents inflammation.

**antimicrobial:** a substance that reduces microbial growth.

**antioxidant:** a substance that inhibits molecular oxidization.

**antiseborrheic:** a substance that helps control the oily secretions produced by the sebaceous glands.

**antiseptic:** a substance that helps control infection.

**antispasmodic:** a substance that helps prevent and relieve muscle spasms and cramping.

**antitussive:** a substance that relieves coughing.

**antiviral:** a substance that combats viral infections.

**aperient:** a substance that relieves constipation.

**aperitif:** a substance that stimulates appetite.

**aphrodisiac:** a substance that enhances sexual libido and improves sexual functioning.

**astringent:** a substance that causes tissues to contract.

**bactericidal:** a substance that kills bacteria.

**calmative:** a substance that acts as a mild sedative.

carminative: a substance that relieves flatulence and facilitates the digestive process.

cephalic: a substance that stimulates the mind or promotes clear thinking.

cholagogue: a substance that stimulates the secretion of bile.

cicatrizant: a substance that promotes healing by encouraging the formation of scar tissue.

cordial: a substance that offers comfort while promoting healing.

cytophylactic: a substance that enhances the body's defense against infection by increasing white blood cell activity.

decongestant: a substance that relieves congestion.

deodorant: a substance that combats body odor.

depurative: a substance that facilitates the removal of toxins from the body and bloodstream.

diaphoretic: a substance that promotes perspiration.

digestive: a substance that promotes normal digestion.

disinfectant: a substance that destroys germs.

diuretic: a substance that removes excess water from the body by promoting urination

emmenagogue: a substance that induces menstruation.

emollient: a substance that softens and soothes skin.

euphoric: a substance that promotes an intense feeling of happiness.

expectorant: a substance that facilitates the expulsion of mucus from the lungs.

febrifuge: a substance that may reduce fever.

fungicide: a substance that kills fungi.

galactagogue: a substance that increases lactation in nursing mothers.

hemostatic: a substance that helps stop bleeding.

hepatic: a substance that acts as a tonic to the liver.

hypertensive: a substance that can elevate blood pressure.

hypnotic: a substance that induces sleep.

hypotensive: a substance that can reduce blood pressure.

insect repellent: a substance that repels insects.

insecticide: a substance that kills insects.

laxative: a substance that induces bowel movements.

nervine: a substance that strengthens and tones the nervous system.

phototoxic: a substance that can increase the risk of sunburn when exposed to direct sunlight after being applied to skin.

relaxant: a substance that encourage relaxation.

rubefacient: a substance that can cause skin to turn red.

sedative: a substance that promotes feelings of tranquility, and that may induce sleep.

stimulant: a substance that enhances alertness.

stomachic: a substance that both enhances appetite and improves digestion.

styptic: a substance that stops external bleeding.

sudorific: a substance that causes sweating.

tonic: a substance that enhances overall well-being.

vasoconstrictor: a substance that can cause blood vessel walls to contract.

vermifuge: a substance that expels intestinal worms.

vulnerary: substance that helps wounds to heal.

# RESOURCES

There are many wonderful aromatherapy resources available. By no means is this an exhaustive list; rather, it is a quick guide to some of the best-known resources. Well-known essential oil brands, comprehensive books on aromatherapy and essential oils, helpful websites, and sources for continuing education are listed here.

## WELL-KNOWN ESSENTIAL OIL BRANDS

**Ancient Ways Botanicals**
Essential oils are available online.

**Aromatics International**
Essential oils are available online.

**Artisan Aromatics**
Essential oils are available online.

**Aura Cacia**
Essential oils are available online and at a variety of retail locations.

**Base Formula Essential Oils & Aromatherapy Sundries**
Essential oils are available online.

**DōTERRA**
Essential oils are sold by independent distributors.

**Dreaming Earth Botanicals**
Essential oils are available online and at a variety of retail locations.

**Edens Garden**
Essential oils are available online.

**Floracopeia**
Essential oils are available online and at a variety of retail locations.

**Healing Solutions**
Essential oils are available online.

**Mountain Rose Herbs**
Essential oils are available online.

**Nature's Bounty**
Essential oils are available online and at a variety of retail locations.

**NOW** (Also known as NOW Foods)
Essential oils are available online and at a variety of retail locations.

**Plant Guru**
Essential oils are available online.

**Plant Therapy**
Essential oils are available online.

**Rocky Mountain Oils**
Essential oils are available online.

**Young Living**
Essential oils are sold by independent distributors.

## BOOKS

*Aromatherapy Workbook* by Marcel Lavabre

*The Art of Aromatherapy: The Healing and Beautifying Properties of the Essential Oils of Flowers and Herbs* by Robert B. Tisserand

*Ayurveda & Aromatherapy: The Earth Essential Guide to Ancient Wisdom and Modern Healing* by Bryan Miller and Light Miller

*The Chemistry of Aromatherapeutic Oils* by E. Joy Bowles

*The Complete Book of Essential Oils and Aromatherapy* by Valerie Ann Worwood

*Essential Oil Maker's Handbook: Extracting, Distilling & Enjoying Plant Essences* by Bettina Malle and Helge Schmickl

*Essential Waters: Hydrosols, Hydrolats & Aromatic Waters* by Marge Clark

*The Fragrant Mind: Aromatherapy for Personality, Mind, Mood and Emotion* by Valerie Ann Worwood

*Gattefossé's Aromatherapy: The First Book on Aromatherapy* by Rene-Maurice Gattefossè and Robert B. Tisserand

*Holistic Aromatherapy for Animals: A Comprehensive Guide to the Use of Essential Oils & Hydrosols with Animals* by Kristen Leigh Bell

*The Illustrated Encyclopedia of Essential Oils* by Julia Lawless

*The Practice of Aromatherapy* by Jean Valnet, MD

*Scents & Scentuality: Essential Oils & Aromatherapy for Romance, Love, and Sex* by Valerie Ann Worwood

## WEBSITES

**Aura Cacia**
Offers a robust online presence, with articles, recipes, essential oils, tools and supplies, and more. www.auracacia.com

**Base Formula Aromatherapy**
Offers a wide range of aromatherapy products, tools, and supplies. www.baseformula.com

**BioSource Naturals**
Carries a full line of aromatherapy supplies and more. www.biosourcenaturals.com

**Floracopeia**

Offers books, free aromatherapy videos, and a wide range of products. www.floracopeia.com

**From Nature With Love**

Provides a vast online library of learning tools along with essential oils, aromatherapy products, and more. www.fromnaturewithlove.com

**Lotus Garden Botanicals**

Offers a wide range of aromatherapy products, an informative blog, and a gift registry. www.lgbotanicals.com

**Mountain Rose Herbs**

Provides an impressive range of essential oils, body care products, packaging, and much more. www.mountainroseherbs.com

**Nature's Gift**

Offers a wide variety of essential oils, aromatherapy products and tools, books, and more. www.naturesgift.com

**Plant Therapy**

Provides daily and monthly specials. The company distinguishes itself with KidSafe, their proprietary line of essential oils and blends for children. Articles, recipes, and other resources for learning are available. www.planttherapy.com

**Somatherapy: Dreaming Earth Botanicals**

Offers an extensive selection of aromatherapy supplies, plus articles and recipes. www.dreamingearth.com

**Starwest Botanicals**

Offers an extensive array of essential oils, aromatherapy supplies, accessories, and more. www.starwest-botanicals.com

# CONTINUING EDUCATION

**Alliance of International Aromatherapists**
www.alliance-aromatherapists.org

**American College of Healthcare Sciences**
www.achs.edu

**Aroma Apothecary Healing Arts Academy**
www.learnaroma.com

**Aromahead Institute**
www.aromahead.com

**Canadian Federation of Aromatherapists**
www.cfacanada.com

**East-West School for Aromatic Studies**
www.theida.com

**Flora Medica**
www.floramedica.com

**Floracopeia**
www.floracopeia.com

**Highlands School of Natural Healing**
www.highlandsnaturalhealing.com

**National Association for Holistic Aromatherapy**
www.naha.org

**Nature's Gift**
www.naturesgift.com

**New York Institute of Aromatherapy**
www.newyorkinstituteofaromatherapy.com

**Pacific Institute of Aromatherapy**
www.newpacificinstituteofaromatherapy.com

**Stillpoint Studies**
www.stillpointstudies.com

**West Coast Institute of Aromatherapy**
www.westcoastaromatherapy.com

# AILMENTS/OILS QUICK REFERENCE

This quick reference guide contains twenty-five of the most common ailments,
along with three suggested essential oils for treating them.

ALLERGIES
chamomile, melissa, peppermint

CONGESTION
cajuput, eucalyptus (all species),
hyssop

CONSTIPATION
anise, black pepper, ginger

CUTS AND SCRAPES
helichrysum, *Eucalyptus
radiata*, lavender

DENTAL PAIN
cajuput, cinnamon leaf,
clove bud

DIGESTIVE COMPLAINTS
peppermint, ginger, Roman
chamomile

EXHAUSTION
black pepper, grapefruit,
mandarin

FLU
bay laurel, clove bud, lemon

HANGOVER
grapefruit, juniper berry,
rosemary

HEADACHE
basil, lavender, melissa

HEARTBURN
German chamomile,
marjoram, peppermint

INSECT BITES
& BEE STINGS
peppermint, spearmint, tea tree

INSECT REPELLENT
citronella, lemongrass, patchouli

INSOMNIA
clary sage, lavender, valerian

IRRITABILITY
mandarin, Roman chamomile,
sandalwood

JET LAG
basil, grapefruit, rosemary

LARYNGITIS
bergamot, cypress, lemon

MENOPAUSE
clary sage, jasmine, vitex berry

MENSTRUAL PROBLEMS
clary sage, marjoram,
vitex berry

MIGRAINE
lavender, peppermint,
Roman chamomile

MUSCLE PAIN
marjoram, oregano, pine

NOSEBLEED
cypress, lavender, lemon

PMS
clary sage, rosemary, vitex berry

SINUSITIS
eucalyptus (all species),
spearmint, tea tree

SUNBURN
eucalyptus (all species),
lavender, Roman chamomile

# REFERENCES

Aromahead Institute. "Component Database." Aromahead.com. Accessed March 18, 2016. components.aromahead.com.

Bartsch, Jennifer, Erik Uhde, and Tunga Salthammer. "Analysis of Odour Compounds from Scented Consumer Products Using Gas Chromatography-Mass Spectrometry and Gas Chromatography-Olfactometry." *Analytica Chimica Acta* 904 (January 2016): 98–106. doi:10.1016/j.aca.2015.11.031.

Basketter, David A., Sylvie Lemoine, and John P. McFadden. "Skin Sensitisation to Fragrance Ingredients: Is There a Role For Household Cleaning/Maintenance Products?" *European Journal of Dermatology* 25, no. 1 (January-February 2015): 7–13. www.ncbi.nlm.nih.gov/pubmed/25547642.

Bouchez, Colette. "Fragrance Allergies: A Sensory Assault." Allergies Health Center, WebMD. Accessed March 17, 2016. www.webmd.com/allergies/features/fragrance-allergies-a-sensory-assault.

Branham, Erin. "The Scent of Love: Ancient Perfumes." *The Getty Iris.* May 1, 2012. blogs.getty.edu/iris/the-scent-of-love-ancient-perfumes.

Bryan, Teresa. "How to Make Essential Oils at Home with Homemade Recipes." *Healthynewage.* Accessed March 18, 2016. www.healthynewage.com/e1.

California College of Ayurveda. "Ayurveda and Aromatherapy: Alternative Medicine for Healing Body-Mind-Spirit." August 6, 2014. Accessed March 17, 2016. www.ayurvedacollege.com/blog/ayurveda-and-aromatherapy-alternative-medicine-healing-body-mind-spirit.

Central Nervous System: Visual Perspectives. "The Thalamus." Accessed March 18, 2016. cnsvp.stanford.edu/atlas/thalamus.html.

Chee, Hee Youn, and Min Hee Lee. "Antifungal Activity of Clove Essential Oil and its Volatile Vapour Against Dermatophytic Fungi." *Mycobiology* 35, no. 4 (December 2007): 241–243. doi:10.4489/MYCO.2007.35.4.241.

Cooksley, Valerie Gennari. *Aromatherapy: A Lifetime Guide to Healing with Essential Oils.* Englewood Cliffs, NJ: Prentice Hall Press, 1996.

Dioscorides. "The Herbal of Dioscorides the Greek: Book One: Aromatics." CancerLynx. Accessed March 17, 2016. www.cancerlynx.com/BOOKONEAROMATICS.PDF.

Edwards, Victoria H. *The Aromatherapy Companion: Medicinal Uses/Ayurvedic Healing/Body-Care Blends/Perfumes & Scents/Emotional Health & Well-Being.* North Adams, MA: Storey Publishing, 1999.

Encyclopedia Britannica. "Avicenna: Persian Philosopher and Scientist." Accessed March 17, 2016. www.britannica.com/biography/Avicenna.

Encyclopedia Britannica. "Enkephalin: Biochemistry." Accessed March 18, 2016. www.britannica.com/science/enkephalin.

Encyclopedia Britannica.com. "Olfactory Bulb: Anatomy." Accessed March 18, 2016. www.britannica.com/science/olfactory-bulb.

Essential Oils Academy. "History of Essential Oils." Accessed March 17, 2016. www.essentialoilsacademy.com/history.

Fordham University, The Jesuit University of New York. "The Life and Works of Hildegard von Bingen (1098–1179)." Accessed March 17, 2016. legacy.fordham.edu/halsall/med/hildegarde.asp.

Friedmann, Terry S., MD, ABHM. "Attention Deficit And Hyperactivity Disorder (ADHD)." Meetup.com. Accessed April 3, 2016. files.meetup.com/1481956 /ADHD%20Research%20by%20Dr.%20Terry %20Friedmann.pdf.

Gattefossé, René-Maurice. *Gattefossé's Aromatherapy: The First Book on Aromatherapy.* Saffron Walden, UK: C.W. Daniel Company, Ltd., 1993.

Gibson, Emma Alvarez. "Best Bets for Beating Gas." Digestive Disorders Health Center, WebMD. Accessed March 25, 2016. www.webmd.com /digestive-disorders/features/embarrassing -conditions.

de Groot, A. C. "Contact Allergy for Perfume Ingredients in Cosmetics and Toilet Articles." *Tijdschrift voor Geneeskunde* 141, no. 12 (March 1997): 571–574. www.ncbi.nlm.nih.gov/pubmed/9190522.

Harman, Ann. *Harvest to Hydrosol: Distill Your Own Exquisite Hydrosols at Home.* Fruitland, WA: botANNicals, 2015.

Healthy Hildegard. "Traditional German Herbal Medicine." Healthy Hildegard.com. Accessed March 17, 2016. www.healthyhildegard.com /traditional-german-herbal-medicine.

History of Medicine Division, U.S. National Library of Medicine. "Greek Medicine: 'I Swear by Apollo Physician . . .': Greek Medicine from the Gods to Galen." Accessed April 5, 2016. www.nlm .nih.gov/hmd/greek/greek_asclepius.html.

History of Medicine Division, U.S. National Library of Medicine. "Greek Medicine: 'I Swear by Apollo Physician . . .': Greek Medicine from the Gods to Galen." Accessed March 17, 2016. www.nlm.nih.gov/hmd/greek/greek_galen.html.

History of Medicine, U.S. National Library of Medicine. "Islamic Culture and the Medical Arts: Al-Razi, the Clinician." Accessed March 17, 2016. www.nlm.nih .gov/exhibition/islamic_medical/islamic_06.html.

Hongratanaworakit, T. "Stimulating Effect of Aromatherapy Massage with Jasmine Oil." *Natural Product Communications* 5, no. 1 (January 2010): 157–162. www.ncbi.nlm.nih.gov/pubmed/20184043.

Keville, Kathi, and Mindy Green. *Aromatherapy: A Complete Guide to the Healing Art.* New York, NY: Crossing Press, 2009.

Lawless, Julia. *The Illustrated Encyclopedia of Essential Oils: The Complete Guide to the Use of Oils in Aromatherapy and Herbalism.* Rockport, MA: Element Books, Inc., 1995.

Levine, Jeffrey M., MD. "Wound Odor: The View from Ancient Greece." Jmlevinemd.com. February 16, 2010. Accessed March 17, 2016. www.jmlevinemd .com/wound-odor-the-view-from-ancient-greece.

Lis-Balchin, Maria. *Aromatherapy Science: A Guide for Healthcare Professionals.* Grayslake, IL: Pharmaceutical Press, 2006.

Lobo, V., A. Patil, A. Phatak, and N. Chandra. "Free Radicals, Antioxidants, and Functional Foods: Impact on Human Health." *Pharmacognosy Reviews* 4, no. 8 (July–December 2010): 118–126. www.ncbi .nlm.nih.gov/pmc/articles/PMC3249911.

Mahler, V. "Contact Allergies in the Elderly." *Der Hautarzt* 66, no. 9 (September 2015): 665–673. doi: 10.1007/s00105-015-3668-z.

Manansala, Paul Kekai. "The Spice Routes." Asiapacificuniverse.com. Accessed April 5, 2016. www.asiapacificuniverse.com/pkm/spiceroutes.htm.

Manniche, Lise. *Sacred Luxuries: Fragrance, Aromatherapy, and Cosmetics in Ancient Egypt.* Ithaca, NY: Cornell University Press, 1999.

National Association for Holistic Aromatherapy. "How Are Essential Oils Extracted?" NAHA.org. Accessed March 18, 2016. www.naha.org/explore -aromatherapy/about-aromatherapy/how-are -essential-oils-extracted.

National Center for Complementary and Integrative Health. "Aromatherapy." Accessed March 17, 2016. https://nccih.nih.gov/health/aromatherapy.

NHR Organic Oils. "New Legislation Concerning Allergens in Essential Oils and Toiletry Products." Accessed March 18, 2016. www.nhrorganicoils.com /frame.php?page=info_21.

Norman, Jeremy. "At Sibudu Cave, the Oldest Known Early Bedding and Use of Medicinal Plants (Circa 75,000 BCE)." History of Information.com. Accessed March 17, 2016. www.historyofinformation.com /expanded.php?id=3465.

Norman, Jeremy. "Probably the Most Beautiful of the Earliest Surviving Scientific Codices (Circa 512)." History of Information.com. May 3, 2014. Accessed March 17, 2016. www.historyofinformation.com /expanded.php?id=1647.

Oils and Plants. "Jean Valnet." Accessed March 17, 2016. www.oilsandplants.com/valnet.htm.

Oils and Plants. "Rene-Maurice Gattefossè." Accessed March 15, 2016. www.oilsandplants.com /gattefosse.htm.

Osborn, David K. "Galen: Greatest Physician of the Roman Empire." Greek Medicine.net. Accessed March 17, 2016. www.greekmedicine.net/whos_who /Galen.html.

Patella, Jessica, ND. "Effects of Rosemary Essential Oil on Mood and Memory." Natural Health Research Institute. Accessed April 5, 2016. www.naturalhealth research.org/rosemary-essential-oil.

PDQ Integrative, Alternative, and Complementary Therapies Editorial Board. "Aromatherapy and Essential Oils (PDQ) Health Professional Version." U.S. National Library of Medicine. Accessed March 17, 2016. www.ncbi.nlm.nih.gov/pubmedhealth /PMH0032645.

PDQ Integrative, Alternative, and Complementary Therapies Editorial Board. "Aromatherapy and Essential Oils (PDQ), Patient Version." U.S. National Library of Medicine. Accessed March 17, 2016. www .ncbi.nlm.nih.gov/pubmedhealth/PMH0032518/.

Price, Shirley. *Aromatherapy Workbook: A Complete Guide to Understanding and Using Essential Oils.* London, UK: Thorsons, 1999.

Roach, John. "Oldest Perfumes Found on 'Aphrodite's Island.'" *National Geographic News.* March 29, 2007. Accessed March 15, 2016. news.nationalgeographic.com /news/2007/03/070329-oldest-perfumes.html.

Salamander Concepts. "The Chemistry of Essential Oils, and Their Chemical Components." Essentialoils .co.za. Accessed March 18, 2016. www.essentialoils .co.za/components.htm.

Sasannejad, P., M. Saeedi, A. Shoeibi, A. Gorji, M. Abbasi, and M. Foroughipour. "Lavender Essential Oil in the Treatment of Migraine Headache: A Place-bo-Controlled Clinical Trial." *European Neurology* 67, no. 5 (2012): 288–291. doi: 10.1159/000335249.

Schnaubelt, Kurt. *Medical Aromatherapy: Healing with Essential Oils.* Berkeley, CA: Frog Books, 1999.

Secret of Thieves. "Four Thieves Vinegar: Evolution of a Medieval Medicine." Accessed March 17, 2016. www.secretofthieves.com/four-thieves-vinegar.cfm.

Shea, Stephen D., Lawrence C. Katz, and Richard Mooney. "Noradrenergic Induction of Odor-Specific Neural Habituation and Olfactory Memories." *The Journal of Neuroscience* 28, no. 42 (October 2008): 10711–10719. doi: 10.1523/JNEUROSCI.3853-08.2008.

The Brunei Times. "Pouches: A Class of Their Own." Bt.com. September 21, 2010. Accessed March 17, 2016. www.bt.com.bn/art-culture/2010/09/21/pouches-class-their-own.

The Chopra Center. "Ayurveda: The Science of Life." Accessed March 17, 2016. www.chopra.com/our-services/ayurveda.

The Middle Ages.net. "The Black Death: Bubonic Plague." Accessed March 17, 2016. www.themiddleages.net/plague.html.

The Robinson Library. "Galen." Accessed March 17, 2016. www.robinsonlibrary.com/medicine/medicine/history/galen.htm.

Thorpe, J. R. "The Strange History of Perfume, from Ancient Roman Foot Fragrance to Napoleon's Cologne." *Bustle*. July 31, 2015. Accessed March 17, 2016. www.bustle.com/articles/101182-the-strange-history-of-perfume-from-ancient-roman-foot-fragrance-to-napoleons-cologne.

Tisserand, Robert. "Safety." Roberttisserand.com. Accessed March 21, 2016. www.roberttisserand.com/category/safety.

Tisserand, Robert B. *The Art of Aromatherapy: The Healing and Beautifying Properties of the Essential Oils of Flowers and Herbs.* Rochester, VT: Healing Arts Press, 1977.

Tisserand, Robert, and Tony Balacs. *Essential Oil Safety: A Guide for Health Care Professionals.* Edinburgh, Scotland: Churchill Livingstone, 1995.

University of Maryland Medical Center. "Aromatherapy." Accessed March 16, 2016. www.umm.edu/health/medical/altmed/treatment/aromatherapy.

Veal, Lowana. "Headlice and Essential Oils." Aromatherapy Global Online Research Archives. August 17. 2011. Accessed March 26, 2016. www.wingedseed.com/Agora/Lice_page.htm.

Verot, Olivier. "The Scent of Opportunity: How China's Fragrance Market Can Reach Its Potential." *Jing Daily*. October 2, 2014. Accessed April 5, 2016. www.jingdaily.com/the-scent-of-opportunity-how-chinas-fragrance-market-can-reach-its-potential/.

White, Gregory Lee. *Essential Oils and Aromatherapy: How to Use Essential Oils for Beauty, Health, and Spirituality.* Detroit, MI: White Willow Books, 2013.

Worwood, Valerie Ann. *The Complete Book of Essential Oils and Aromatherapy:* Novato, CA: New World Library, 1991.

Worwood, Valerie Ann. *The Fragrant Mind: Aromatherapy for Personality, Mind, Mood, and Emotion.* Novato, CA: New World Library, 1996.

# OILS INDEX

# RECITE INDEX

## HOME RECIPES

# GENERAL INDEX

# ABOUT THE AUTHOR

ANNE KENNEDY began her lifelong study of herbs and plants as a child in Montana's Bitterroot Valley, starting with an interest in Native American herbal remedies. Today she is a writer who specializes in a wide variety of natural health, gardening, and sustainability topics. She has written several books on essential oils and herbal medicine, including *The Portable Essential Oils* (2016), *Essential Oils Natural Remedies* (2015), and *Essential Oils for Beginners* (2013). Self-sufficiency, an active outdoor lifestyle, and a strong focus on the interconnectedness of body, mind, and spirit serve as her inspiration and her cornerstone for healthy living. Anne lives and works from her home on a small organic farm in the mountains of West Virginia. Her favorite essential oil is frankincense.

CPSIA information can be obtained
at www.ICGtesting.com
Printed in the USA
BVOW07s0342270616

453411BV00003BC/4/P